everyday
fresh
MEALS IN MINUTES

Photography by Con Poulos

EVERYDAY FRESH
Copyright © Donna Hay Pty Ltd 2020
Design copyright © Donna Hay Pty Ltd 2020
Photography copyright © Con Poulos 2020
Recipes and styling: Donna Hay
Art direction and design: Genevieve McKelvey
Senior designer: Hannah Schubert
Copy editor: Daniela Bertollo
Recipe testing: Peta Dent, Sarah Watson, Madeleine Jeffreys, Sandy Goh and Melissa Burge.

Fourth Estate
An imprint of HarperCollins*Publishers*

HarperCollins*Publishers*
Australia • Brazil • Canada • France • Germany • Holland • Hungary
India • Italy • Japan • Mexico • New Zealand • Poland • Spain • Sweden
Switzerland • United Kingdom • United States of America

First published in Australia in 2020
by HarperCollins*Publishers* Australia Pty Limited
Level 13, 201 Elizabeth Street, Sydney NSW 2000
ABN 36 009 913 517
harpercollins.com.au

A catalogue record for this book is available from the National Library of Australia
ISBN 978 1 4607 5812 0

Reproduction by Splitting Image
Printed and bound in China by 1010 Printing International Limited on 140gsm Golden Sun Woodfree
6 5 4 3 2 1   20 21 22 23

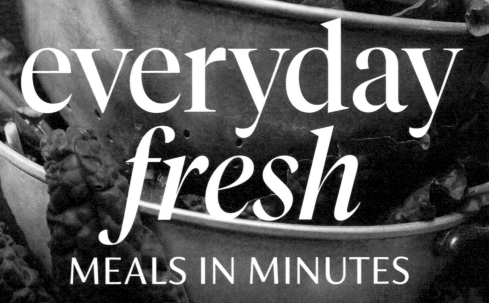

everyday *fresh*

MEALS IN MINUTES

FOURTH ESTATE

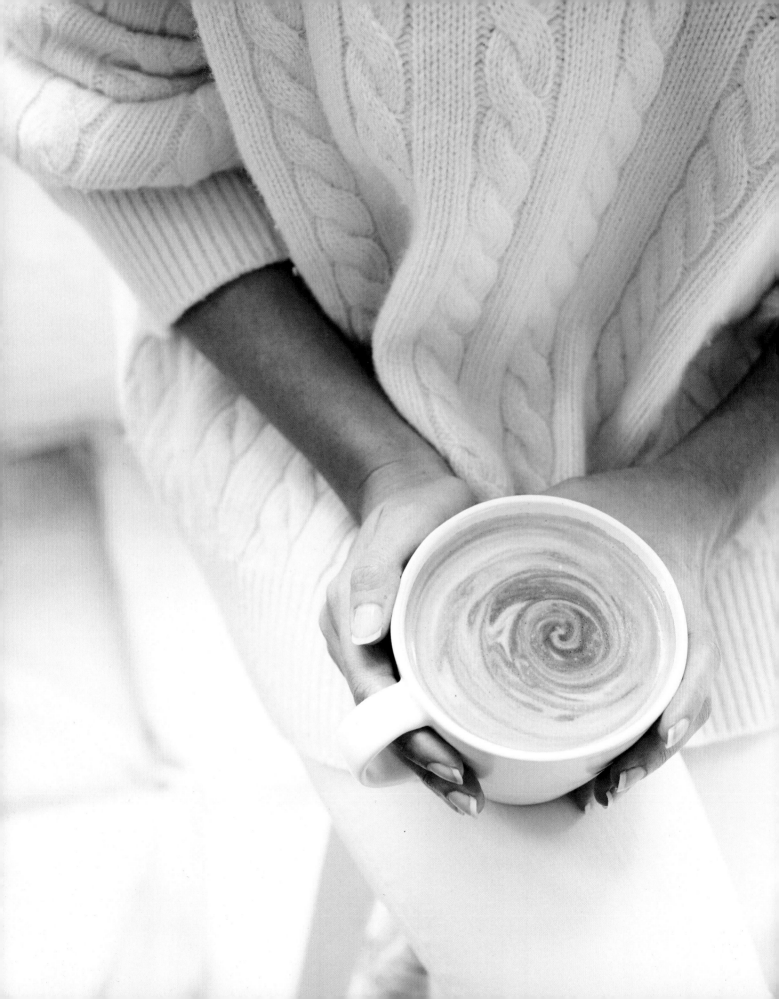

contents

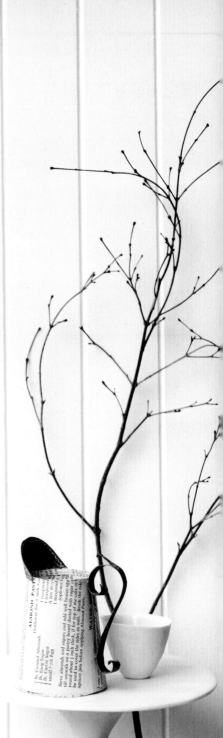

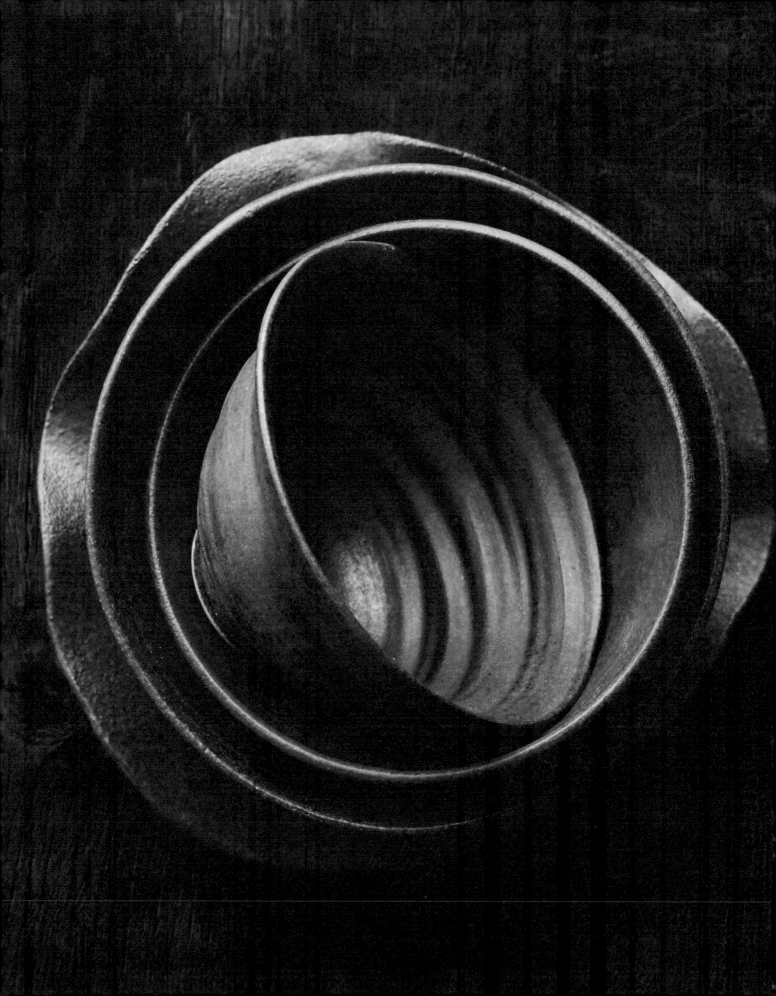

watch
cook · *learn* · love

Find delicious inspiration
as you WATCH RECIPES from
everyday fresh be brought to life.

Come visit me at
www.donnahay.com/video

introduction

One of the questions I get asked most frequently is if I still cook at home. The answer is yes. *Absolutely.* So I'm constantly on the lookout for ways to make a classic EASIER, QUICKER and BETTER FOR YOU, as long as it still *tastes amazingly good.*

We all want to create delicious meals with a minimum of fuss. When you add *healthy or nutritious* to that, some people shy away... concerned that a nutritional boost will be at the expense of flavour and ease. But I say *never!*

If I can create an almost-instant dinner or a quick one-pan dish that makes someone feel great because it's super delicious, is NUTRITIONALLY UPSCALED with better-for-you ingredients, or that helps them bring *a little more balance to their life* – that's success!

I hope these recipes inspire you to *a new level of nourishing yum.*

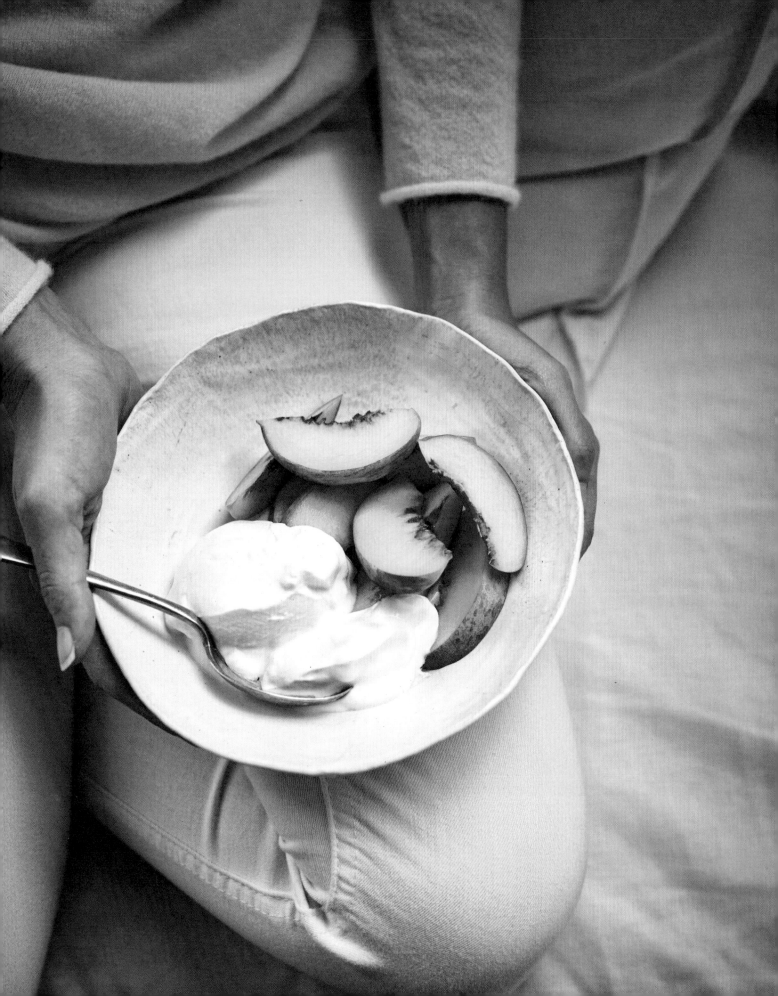

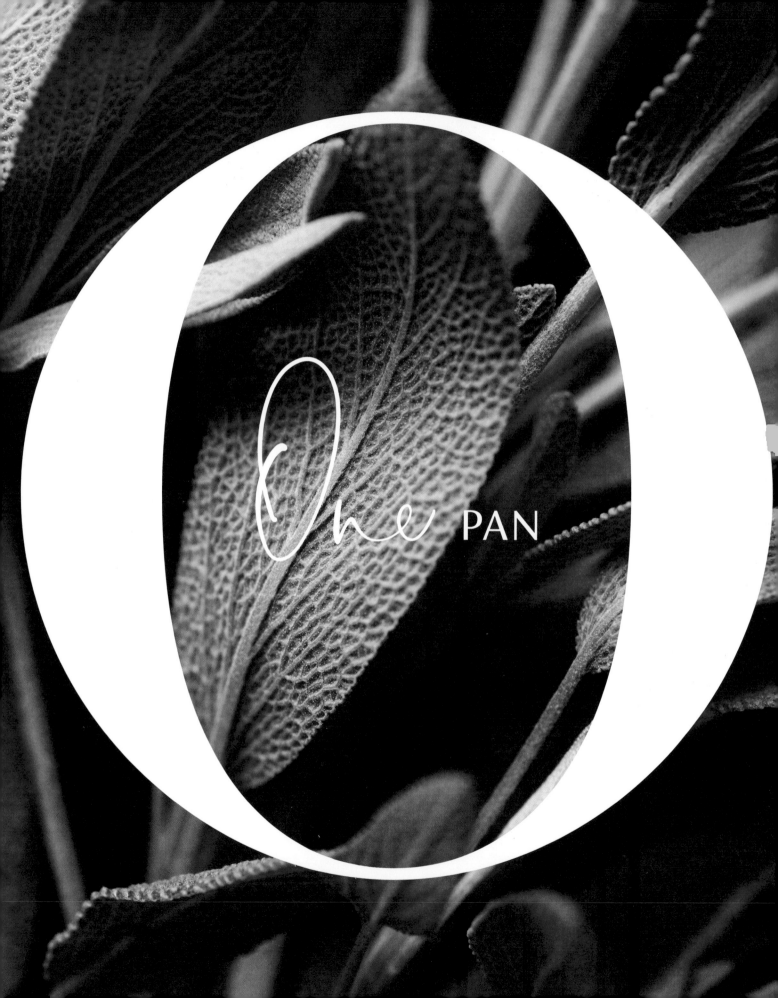

One PAN

If I'm honest, the only thing I like more than an EFFORTLESS DINNER, is when the clean-up is a breeze. These one-pan wonder recipes ensure all the GOODNESS AND FABULOUS FLAVOUR *stays in one dish*. Keeping the process and delivery uncomplicated is a comforting remedy to life's hustle and bustle. *A recipe for success!*

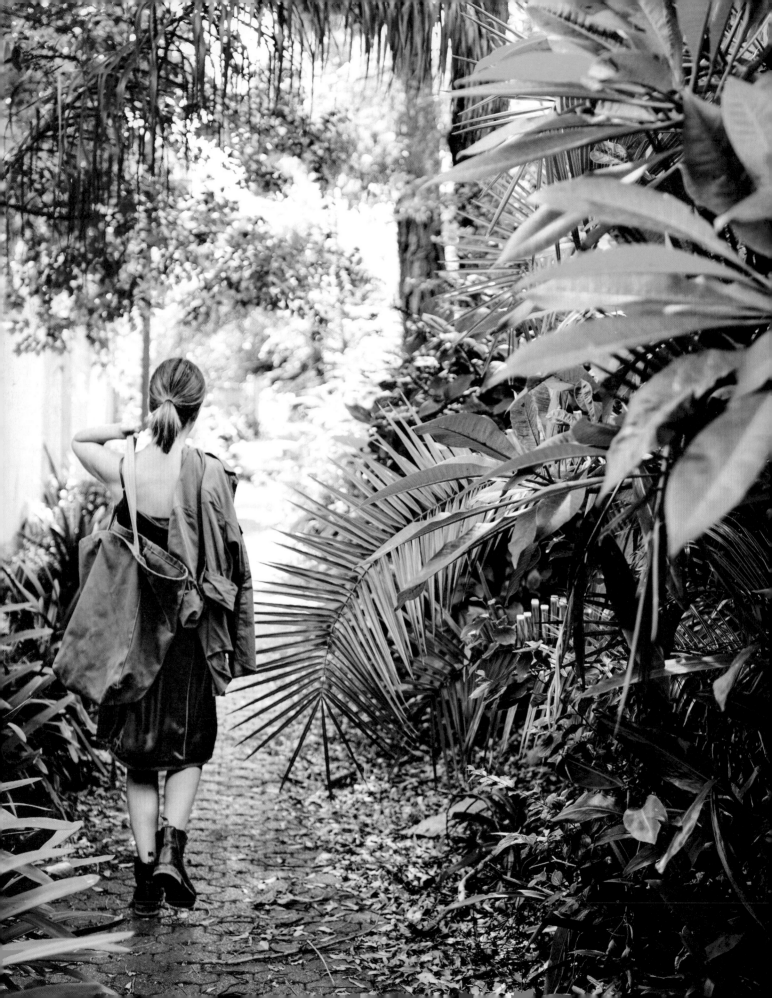

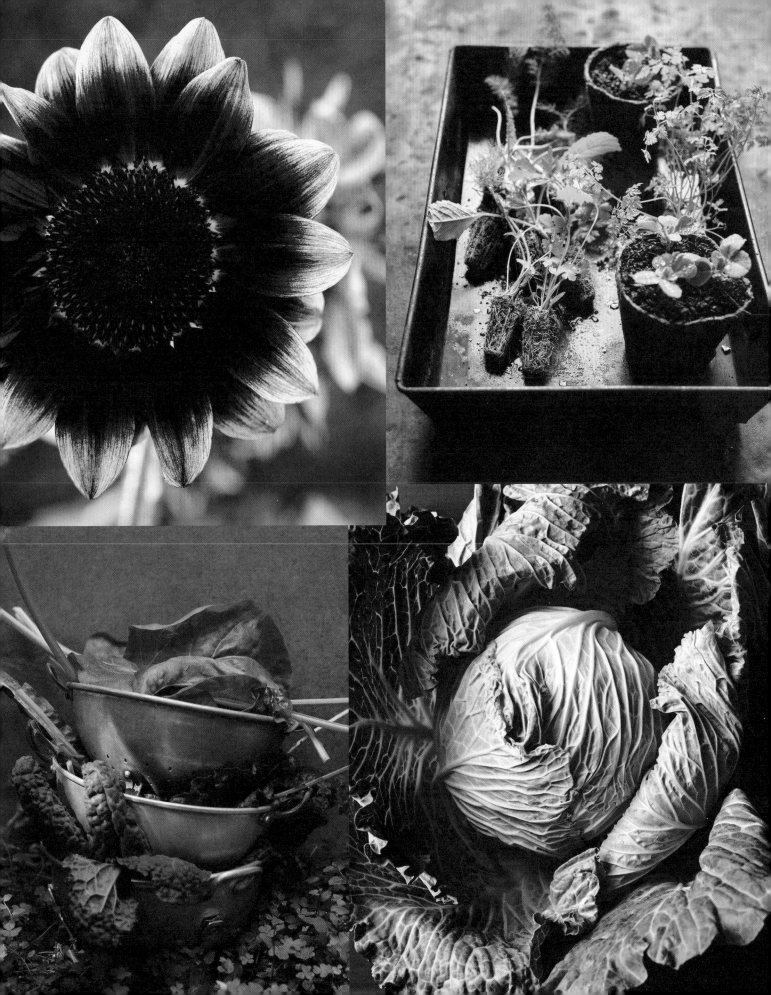

sticky SOY CHICKEN with *sesame noodles*

1 tablespoon light-flavoured extra virgin olive oil
150g (5¼ oz) dried soba noodles, cooked
2 zucchini (courgettes), shredded using a julienne peeler
2 tablespoons white or black sesame seeds
coriander (cilantro) leaves, to serve
chicken meatballs
600g (1 lb ¼ oz) chicken mince
¼ cup (50g/1¾ oz) white chia seeds
2 cloves garlic, crushed
2 tablespoons finely grated ginger
2 tablespoons hoisin sauce
1 large green chilli, finely chopped
2 green onions (scallions), finely chopped
sticky soy sauce
½ cup (125ml/4¼ fl oz) soy sauce
1 tablespoon white miso paste (shiro)
¾ cup (180ml/6 fl oz) mirin (Japanese rice wine)
1 tablespoon sesame oil
2 tablespoons rice wine vinegar
¼ cup (90g/3 oz) honey

Preheat oven to 220°C (425°F).

To make the chicken meatballs, place the chicken, chia seeds, garlic, ginger, hoisin, chilli and onion in a bowl and mix to combine. Roll heaped tablespoons of the mixture into balls, place on a tray lined with baking paper and set aside.

Pour the oil onto a large deep-sided baking tray. Bake for 5 minutes or until hot. Add the meatballs to the tray and bake for 5 minutes.

To make the sticky soy sauce, whisk together the soy, miso, mirin, sesame oil, vinegar and honey. Remove the meatballs from the oven and carefully pour the soy mixture over the meatballs. Return to the oven and bake for 15 minutes or until the meatballs are cooked through and the pan sauce is thickened.

To serve, place noodles and zucchini into serving bowls and sprinkle with sesame. Top with meatballs, sticky soy sauce and coriander.

SERVES 4

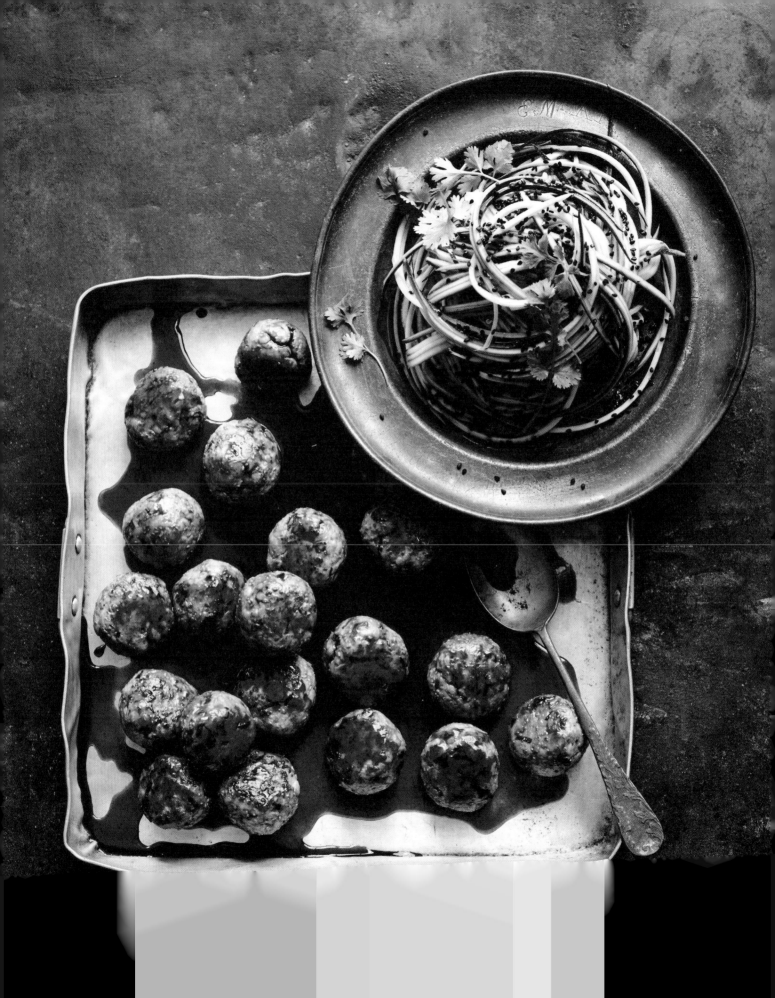

maple AND chilli roasted pumpkin *with quinoa tabouli*

1 x 2kg (4 lb 4 oz) or 2 x 1kg (2 lb 3 oz) butternut pumpkin
  (squash), halved
2 tablespoons extra virgin olive oil
1 tablespoon pure maple syrup
1 teaspoon chilli flakes
sea salt and cracked black pepper
¼ cup (40g/1½ oz) roasted almonds, chopped
quinoa tabouli
2 cups (320g/11¼ oz) cooked quinoa
½ cup (8g/¼ oz) torn mint leaves
60g (2 oz) wild rocket (arugula) leaves
lemon tahini dressing
½ cup (140g/5 oz) hulled tahini
⅔ cup (160ml/5½ fl oz) lemon juice
1 cup (250ml/8½ fl oz) water
1 clove garlic, crushed
sea salt flakes

Preheat oven to 220°C (425°F).

Scoop the seeds from the pumpkin and discard. Place pumpkin, cut side up, onto a baking tray. Using the tip of a sharp knife, make some shallow slashes into the pumpkin flesh. Combine the oil, maple, chilli, salt and pepper and brush over the pumpkin. Cover with aluminium foil and roast for 20 minutes. Remove the foil and roast for a further 40 minutes or until the pumpkin is golden and soft.

To make the quinoa tabouli, in a large bowl combine the quinoa, mint, and rocket.

To make the lemon tahini dressing, in a small bowl, place the tahini, lemon juice, water, garlic and salt. Mix to combine.

To serve, place the pumpkin onto a serving platter and top with the tabouli. Drizzle with the lemon tahini dressing and sprinkle over almonds. **SERVES 4**

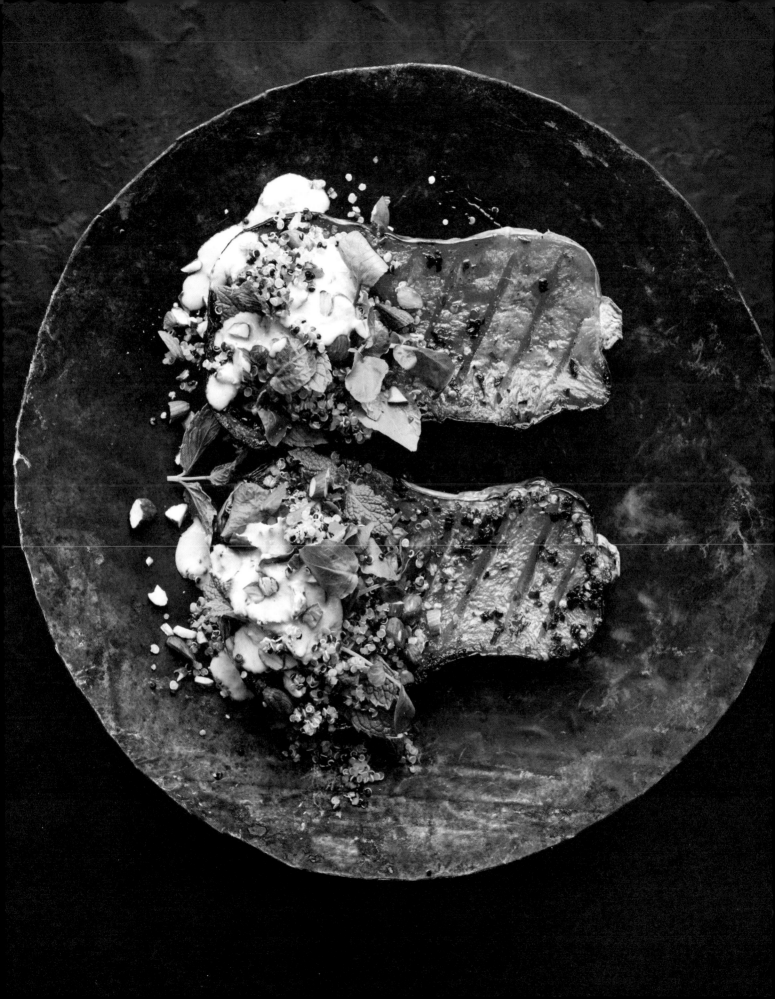

super GREEN baked *risotto*

1 tablespoon extra virgin olive oil
1 leek, sliced
2 tablespoons lemon thyme leaves
sea salt and cracked black pepper
1½ cups (300g/10½ oz) arborio rice
4½ cups (1.25 litres/42 fl oz) vegetable or chicken stock
100g (3½ oz) baby spinach leaves
4 cups (120g/4¼ oz) shredded kale leaves (stems removed)
2 teaspoons finely grated lemon rind
1 tablespoon lemon juice
¼ cup (5g/⅛ oz) roughly chopped basil leaves
½ cup (40g/1½ oz) finely grated parmesan

Preheat oven to 180°C (350°F).

Heat a large deep ovenproof frying pan or flameproof roasting pan over medium heat. Add the oil, leek, lemon thyme, salt and pepper and cook for 5 minutes or until leek is golden and soft.

Add the rice and stock and stir to combine. Cover with a tight-fitting lid or sheets of aluminium foil and bake in the oven for 20 minutes. Allow to stand covered for 5 minutes.

Remove the lid and stir the spinach, kale, lemon rind and juice into the risotto. Continue stirring until risotto is creamy and the greens are tender. Stir through the basil and parmesan and serve. **SERVES 4**

I love this NO-FUSS, no-stir risotto. It's *the perfect base to get creative with* – try swapping out the kale for finely chopped broccoli or go SUPER SIMPLE by scattering in some frozen peas. *The choice is yours!*

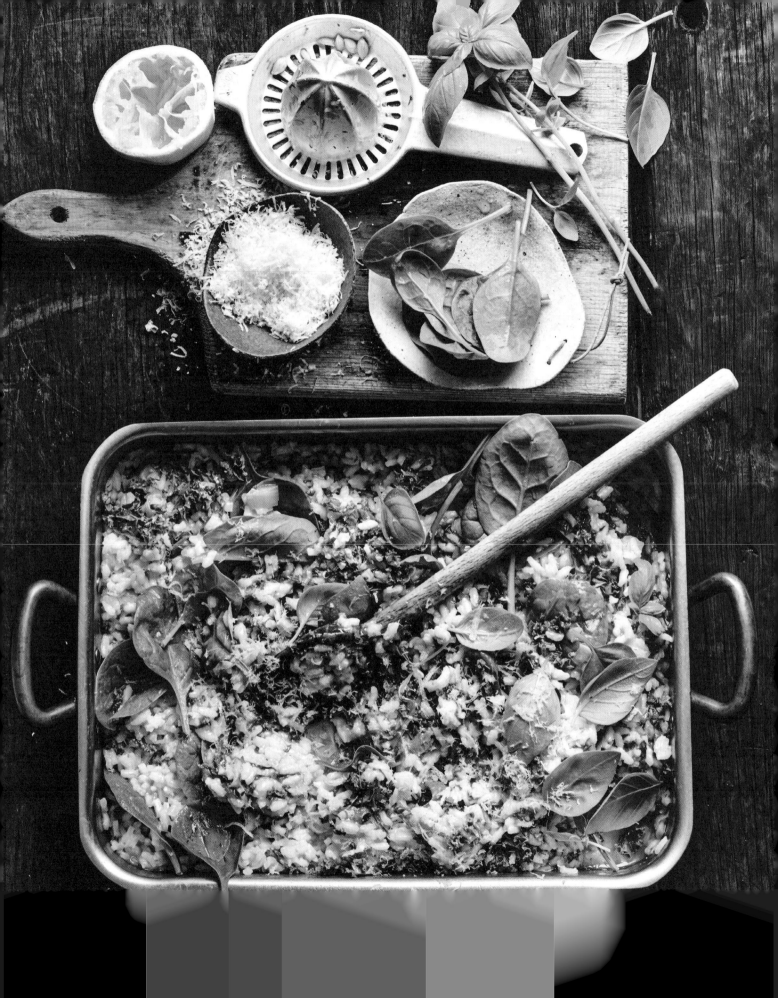

parmesan AND quinoa eggplant schnitzels

2 x 350g (12¼ oz) medium eggplants (aubergines), trimmed and
  sliced lengthways into 1.5cm (½ inch) thick slices
sea salt flakes
1½ cups (150g/5¼ oz) quinoa flakes
½ cup (40g/1½ oz) finely grated parmesan
cracked black pepper
2 eggs, lightly beaten
extra virgin olive oil, for drizzling
500g (1 lb 1 oz) vine-ripened cherry tomatoes
rocket (arugula) leaves, fresh mozzarella and basil leaves, to serve

Preheat oven to 220°C (425°F).
  Sprinkle both sides of eggplant slices with a little salt and allow
to stand for 10 minutes. Drain away excess liquid and pat dry.
  Combine the quinoa, parmesan and pepper in a shallow bowl.
  Dip the eggplant into the egg, then press both sides into the
quinoa mixture.
  Place the eggplant on a large baking tray lined with non-stick baking
paper and drizzle generously with oil. Add the tomatoes to the tray.
Roast for 25–30 minutes or until the eggplant is golden and crisp.
  To serve, place the eggplant and tomatoes onto serving plates.
Serve with rocket, mozzarella and basil. **SERVES 4**

I've used quinoa here because it makes *such a great schnitzel crumb.* It's a SUPER-CRUNCHY and gluten-free *alternative to breadcrumbs* and, as a bonus, quinoa is loaded with all the GOOD STUFF.

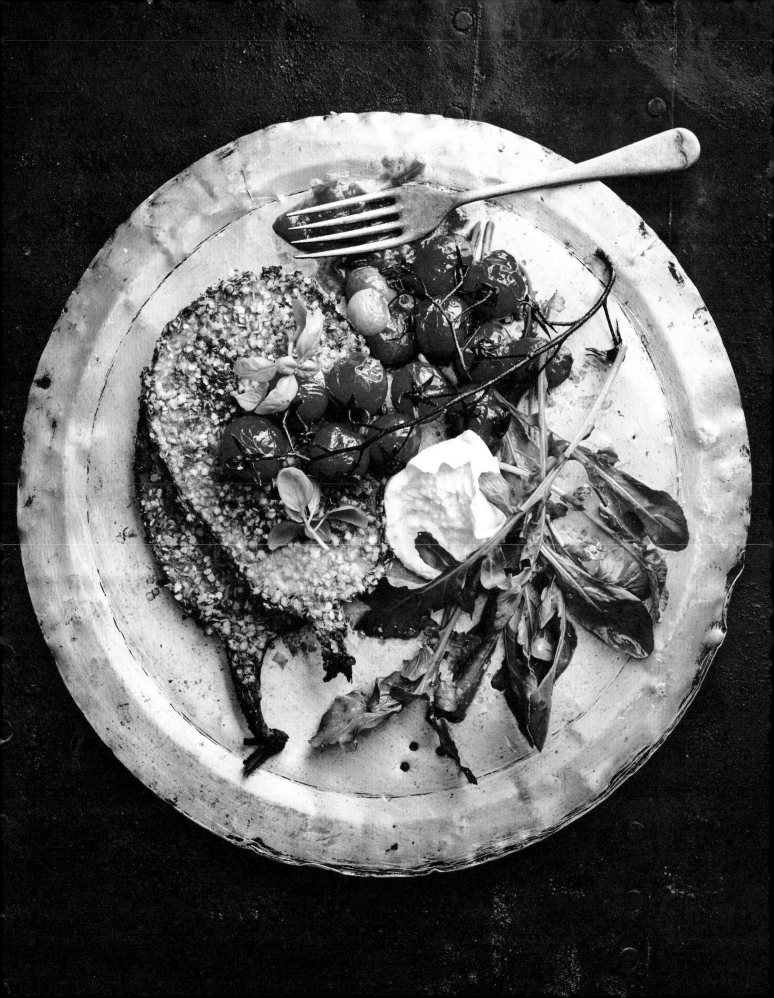

lemon, OLIVE AND butter bean *chicken*

¼ cup (60ml/2 fl oz) extra virgin olive oil
2 lemons, thickly sliced
8 cloves garlic, skin on, crushed
¾ cup (45g/1½ oz) green Sicilian olives
12 sprigs oregano or marjoram
sea salt and cracked black pepper
4 x 150g (5¼ oz) chicken breast fillets (4 small), trimmed
1 x 400g (14 oz) can butter beans (lima beans), drained, rinsed
12 small stalks cavolo nero (Tuscan kale), stems removed

Preheat oven to 200°C (400°F).

Place the oil, lemon, garlic, olives, oregano, salt and pepper in a
large roasting pan lined with non-stick baking paper. Toss to combine.
Bake for 10 minutes then add the chicken and butter beans. Coat the
chicken in the pan juices and bake for 10 minutes. Add the cavolo nero
to the pan and bake for a further 5 minutes or until the cavolo nero
is crisp and the chicken is cooked through.

To serve, slice the chicken into thick slices and place onto serving
plates with the crispy cavolo nero, beans, olives and pan juices. **SERVES 4**

For a dish that is filled with PUNCHY FLAVOURS
and textures, this chicken dish takes *surprisingly
little effort* to make. The lemon, garlic, salty olives,
creamy beans and crispy cavolo nero do all the heavy
lifting. It's what I call ONE-PAN PERFECT!

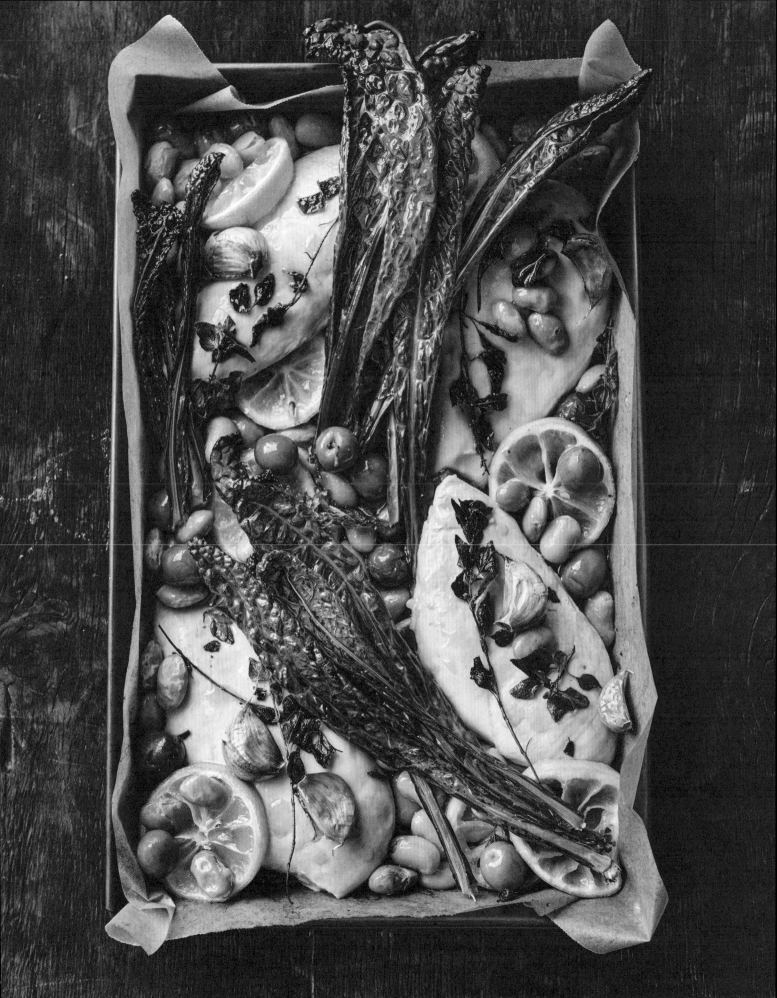

caramelised CABBAGE
with beetroot *and feta salad*

1 medium green cabbage, sliced into 2.5cm (1 inch) thick steaks
2 tablespoons extra virgin olive oil
sea salt and cracked black pepper
3 medium (300g/10½ oz) beetroot, scrubbed and thinly sliced
½ cup (125ml/4¼ oz) balsamic vinegar
1 tablespoon brown sugar
½ teaspoon sea salt flakes
200g (7 oz) firm feta, sliced
½ cup (12g/½ oz) dill leaves
½ cup (12g/½ oz) flat-leaf parsley leaves

Preheat oven to 220°C (425°F).
  Place cabbage on a large baking tray lined with non-stick baking paper. Brush with oil, season with salt and pepper and cover with foil. Roast for 20 minutes. Remove foil and roast for a further 25 minutes or until charred and caramelised.
  While the cabbage is cooking, place beetroot in a bowl with vinegar, sugar and salt. Mix to combine.
  Top cabbage with beetroot, feta, dill and parsley. Drizzle with beetroot pickling liquid to serve. **SERVES 4**

Cooked to a CARAMELISED deep golden brown, this is *my absolute favourite way* to eat cabbage. Charring cabbage takes it to a *whole new level of deliciousness.* Fresh beetroot and herbs add a BRIGHT balance of flavour.

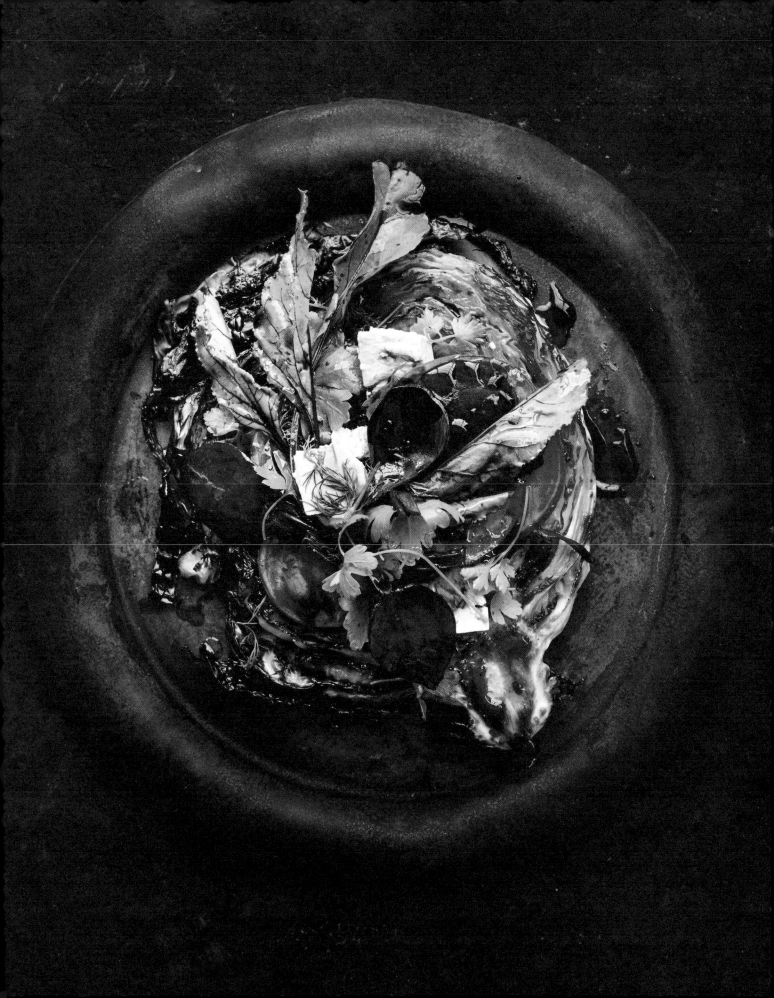

oven baked KALE GNOCCHI
with *balsamic tomatoes*

3 x 400g (14 oz) cans cherry tomatoes
2 tablespoons balsamic vinegar
4 cloves garlic, sliced
2 basil stalks
2 cups (500ml/17 fl oz) chicken or vegetable stock
sea salt and cracked black pepper
1 tablespoon extra virgin olive oil
finely grated parmesan and basil leaves, to serve
kale gnocchi
4 cups (120g/4 oz) finely shredded kale leaves, blanched,
  well drained
2 teaspoons finely grated lemon rind
1 cup (80g/2¾ oz) finely grated parmesan
2 cups (480g/1 lb) fresh ricotta
2 tablespoons finely chopped flat-leaf parsley leaves
⅔ cup (100g/3½ oz) brown rice flour, sifted, plus extra for dusting
sea salt and cracked black pepper

Preheat oven to 220°C (425°F).
  Place the tomatoes, balsamic, garlic, basil stalks, stock, salt and
pepper in a large deep-sided roasting tray. Cover with aluminium foil
and bake for 20 minutes or until the sauce is simmering.
  To make the gnocchi, place the kale, lemon rind, parmesan, ricotta,
parsley, flour, salt and pepper in a large bowl and mix to combine
(this mixture should be a little sticky).
  Divide the gnocchi mixture into 4 pieces and press out each on
a lightly floured board into a 30cm (12 inch) log. Cut each log into
4cm (1½ inch) pieces, gently pressing into shape and set aside.
  Add the gnocchi to the simmering balsamic tomatoes, drizzle with
the oil and bake, uncovered, for a further 15 minutes or until the
gnocchi are cooked through.
  To serve, ladle gnocchi and tomatoes into bowls and sprinkle with
parmesan and basil leaves. **SERVES 4-6**

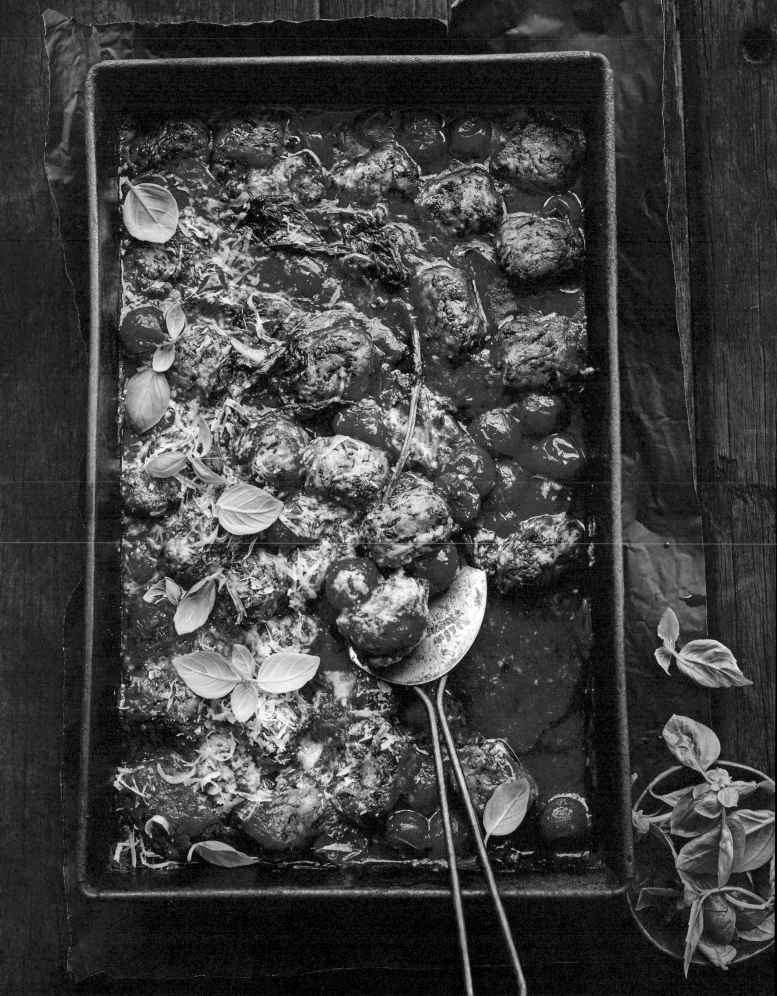

carrot AND kimchi fritters with chilli egg

500g (1 lb 1 oz) carrots, peeled and shredded using a julienne peeler
1½ cups (200g/7 oz) grated cauliflower
1 cup (280g/10 oz) kimchi, shredded
4 eggs, lightly whisked
¼ cup (60ml/2 fl oz) milk
⅓ cup (55g/2 oz) brown rice flour
2 tablespoons white chia seeds
extra virgin olive oil, for cooking
green snake beans, blanched
green onion (scallion), thinly sliced, chilli sauce and
   purple shiso leaves, to serve
chilli eggs
1 tablespoon extra virgin olive oil
2 red chillies, finely sliced
1 teaspoon finely grated ginger
4 eggs

To make the fritters, place the carrot, cauliflower, kimchi, eggs, milk, flour and chia in a bowl and mix to combine.

Heat 2 medium non-stick frying pans over medium heat. Add a little oil and 1 cupful of mixture into each pan. Spread the mixture thinly to cover the base of the pan and cook for 5-7 minutes each side or until golden. Repeat with remaining mixture, adding more oil as necessary to make each fritter. Keep warm until ready to serve.

To make the chilli eggs, return frying pans to medium heat and add a teaspoon of oil to each.

Sprinkle each pan with chilli and ginger and cook for 1-2 minutes. Add 1 egg, lightly whisked, to each pan and swirl to the edges. Cook for 3-4 minutes or until edges are crisp. Remove to a board and roll thinly. Repeat to make 4 chilli egg omelettes. Thinly slice omelettes.

To serve, divide fritters between plates, top with beans, chilli eggs, green onion, chilli sauce and purple shiso. **SERVES 4**

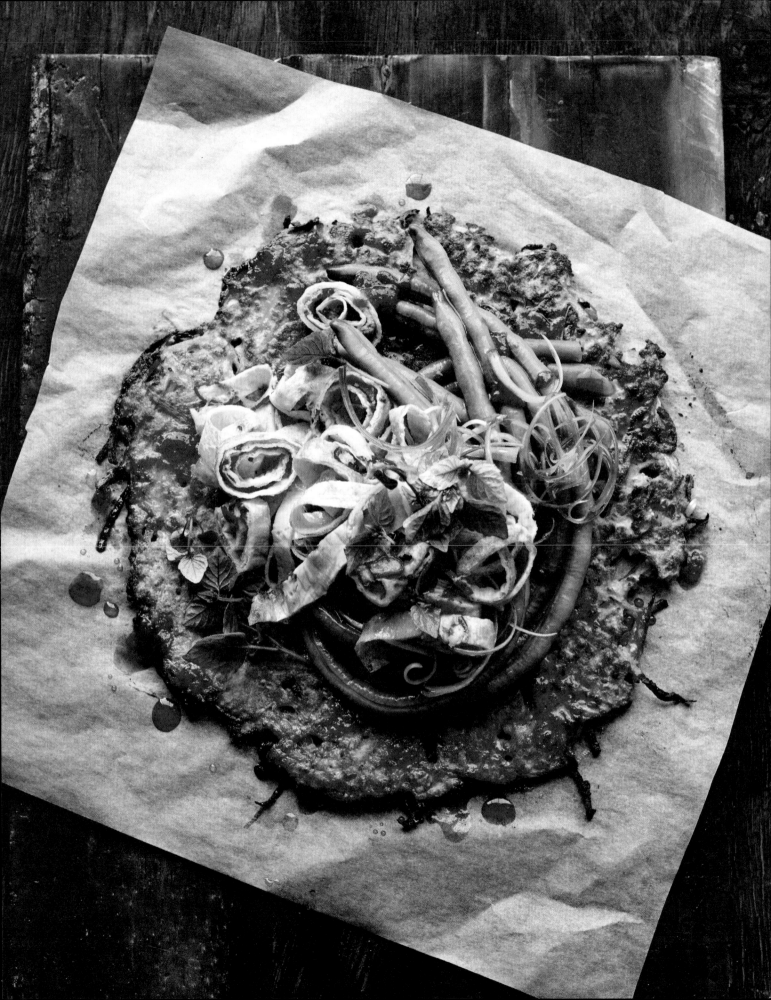

super GREEN **reuben**

2 tablespoons extra virgin olive oil, plus extra to brush
2 cloves garlic, sliced
2 tablespoons roughly chopped oregano leaves
6 cups (180g/6¼ oz) roughly chopped kale (stems removed)
300g (10½ oz) baby spinach leaves
2 tablespoons chopped dill
125g (4½ oz) cream cheese
1 tablespoon horseradish cream
1¼ cups (150g/5¼ oz) sauerkraut, drained
sea salt and cracked black pepper
8 slices rye or wholemeal (whole-wheat) bread
4 large slices Swiss cheese
dill pickles, to serve

Heat a large non-stick frying pan over medium-high heat.
Add the oil, garlic and oregano and cook for 2 minutes or until soft.
Add the kale in batches and cook, stirring, for 5 minutes or until wilted.
Add the spinach, dill, cream cheese, horseradish and sauerkraut
to the pan and stir for 2 minutes or until spinach is wilted and the
ingredients are combined. Season with salt and pepper.
Pile the kale mixture onto 4 slices of the bread and top with the
cheese and remaining bread slices.
Wipe out the pan and place over medium heat. Brush the bread with
the extra oil and cook for 4 minutes each side or until the bread is well
toasted and the cheese is melted. Serve with pickles. **SERVES 4**

I love *bringing balance to a guilty pleasure*, like
this Reuben. Here's your chance to enjoy the
most delicious CRUNCHY and *cheesy toasted
sandwich* while still looking after yourself with
a good dose of NOURISHING GREENS.

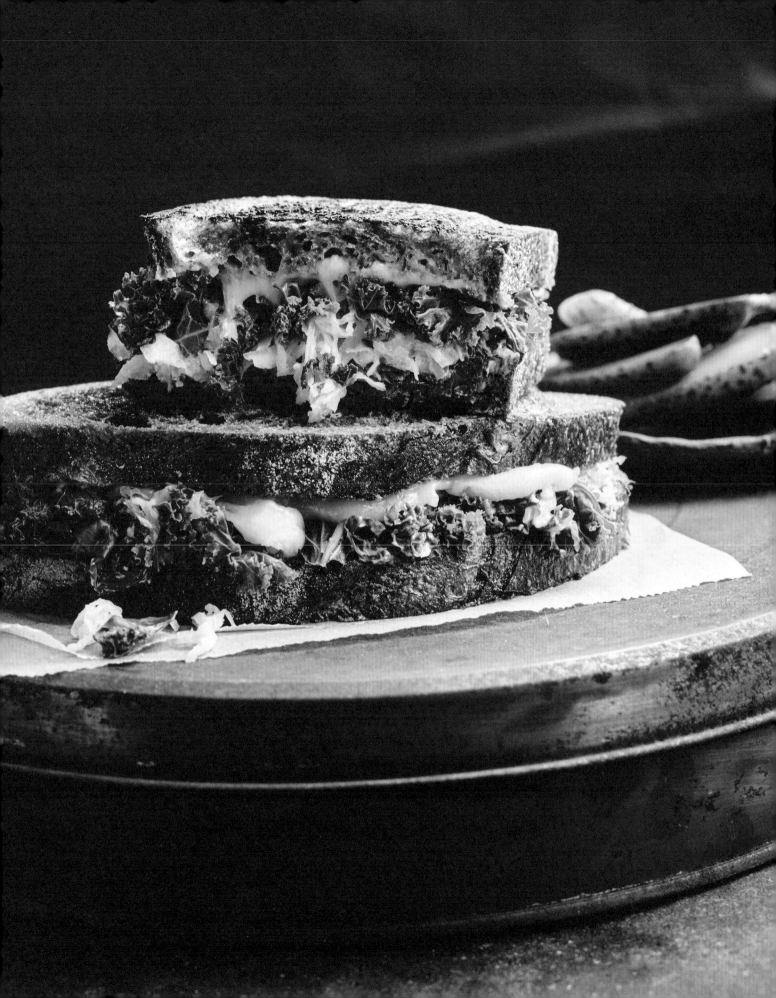

minted LAMB, eggplant, and *feta pie*

3 x 350g (12¼ oz) medium eggplants (aubergines), thinly sliced
  into rounds
500g (1 lb 1 oz) lamb mince (good-quality lean mince)
1 cup (70g/2½ oz) fresh wholemeal (whole-wheat) breadcrumbs
2 tablespoons honey
2 teaspoons ground cumin
¼ cup (4g/¼ oz) chopped mint leaves, plus extra
  mint leaves to serve
2 tablespoons pine nuts
sea salt and cracked black pepper
150g (5¼ oz) firm feta
8 oregano sprigs
1 teaspoon sumac
extra virgin olive oil, for drizzling
minted yoghurt
1 cup (280g/10 oz) plain Greek-style (thick) yoghurt
2 tablespoons shredded mint leaves
sea salt flakes

Preheat oven to 180°C (350°F).

Brush a 28cm (11 inch) round baking dish with oil. Layer half the
eggplant in a circular motion on the baking dish, starting from the
centre and working your way out.

Place the mince, breadcrumbs, honey, cumin, mint and pine nuts in
a large bowl with salt and pepper and mix to combine.

Press mince onto eggplant and crumble over the feta. Add another
layer of eggplant starting from the centre and working your way out.
Sprinkle over oregano sprigs and top with sumac and drizzle with oil.

Bake for 40-45 minutes or until the lamb is cooked through and the
eggplant is golden.

While the pie is cooking, make the minted yoghurt. Add yoghurt,
mint and salt to taste to a bowl and mix to combine.

To serve, divide pie between plates and top with minted yoghurt
and extra mint. **SERVES 4**

It's a pie but not as you know it. I've taken CLASSIC
Greek ingredients and recreated them into this
layered creation that makes each flavour really
SHINE. It's *impressively tasty with minimal effort.*

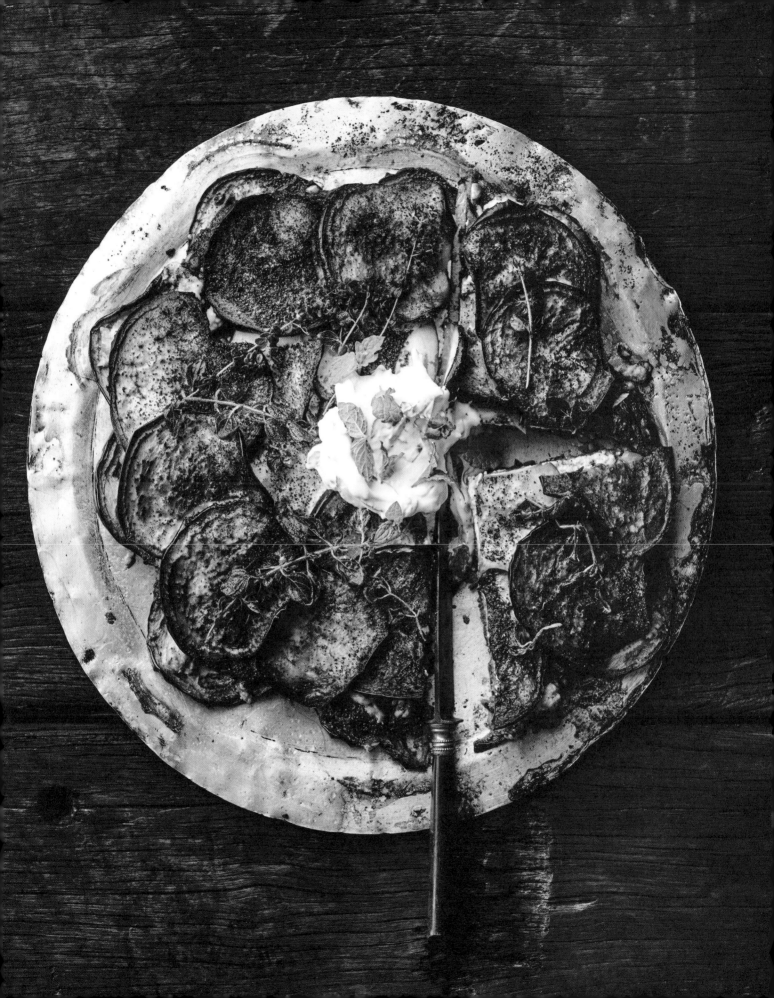

Almost
INSTANT DINNERS

When there's barely time to eat dinner, let alone make it, you need speedy solutions – FRESH FOOD, IN AN INSTANT, *that delivers on taste as well as speed*. These recipes call upon the HEROES IN YOUR PANTRY, lifted to new heights with a flutter of fresh vegies, herbs and spices to *make a meal for two in, literally, minutes.*

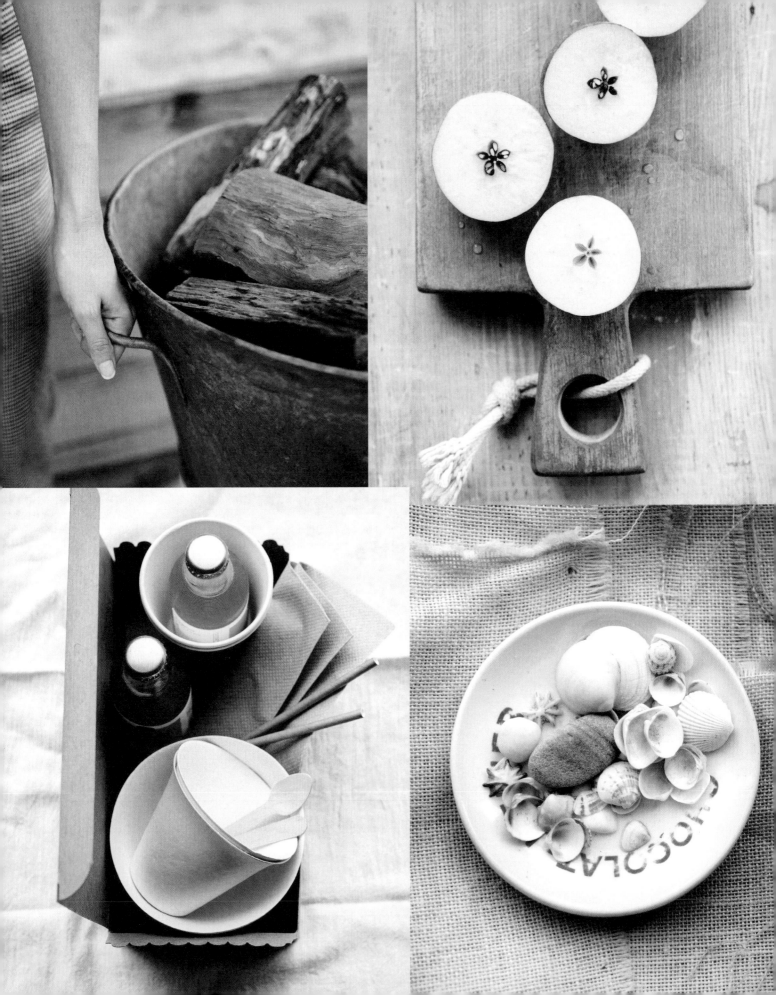

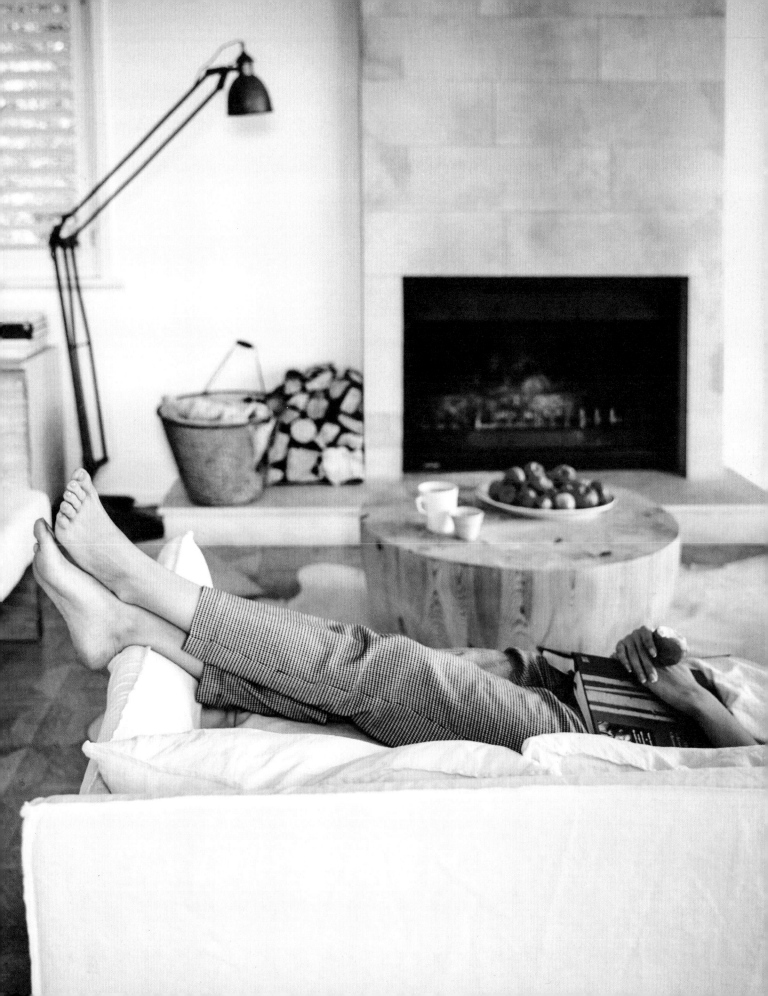

pasta WITH GARLIC CRUMBS, lemon *and ricotta*

200g (7 oz) dried wholemeal (whole-wheat) spaghetti or linguine
2 tablespoons extra virgin olive oil, plus extra for drizzling
2 cloves garlic, sliced
2 slices sourdough bread, torn into small pieces (crusts on)
1 tablespoon shredded lemon rind
4 white anchovy fillets, finely chopped (optional)
¼ cup (6g/¼ oz) torn flat-leaf parsley leaves
30g (1 oz) wild rocket (arugula) leaves
½ cup (120g/4¼ oz) fresh ricotta
finely grated parmesan and lemon wedges (optional), to serve

Cook the pasta in a large saucepan of boiling salted water for
8 minutes or until al dente. Drain and set aside.

Return saucepan to medium-low heat. Add the oil, garlic and bread
and toss until golden. Add lemon rind, anchovy, pasta, parsley and
rocket and toss to coat.

To serve, divide pasta between bowls and top with ricotta. Drizzle
with extra oil, sprinkle with parmesan and serve with lemon wedges,
if you like. **SERVES 2**

THE SIMPLICITY of this dish is fantastic and
the *balance of flavours will surprise you.* If you don't
want to use anchovies, that's fine. Replace them
with SALTY CAPERS instead.

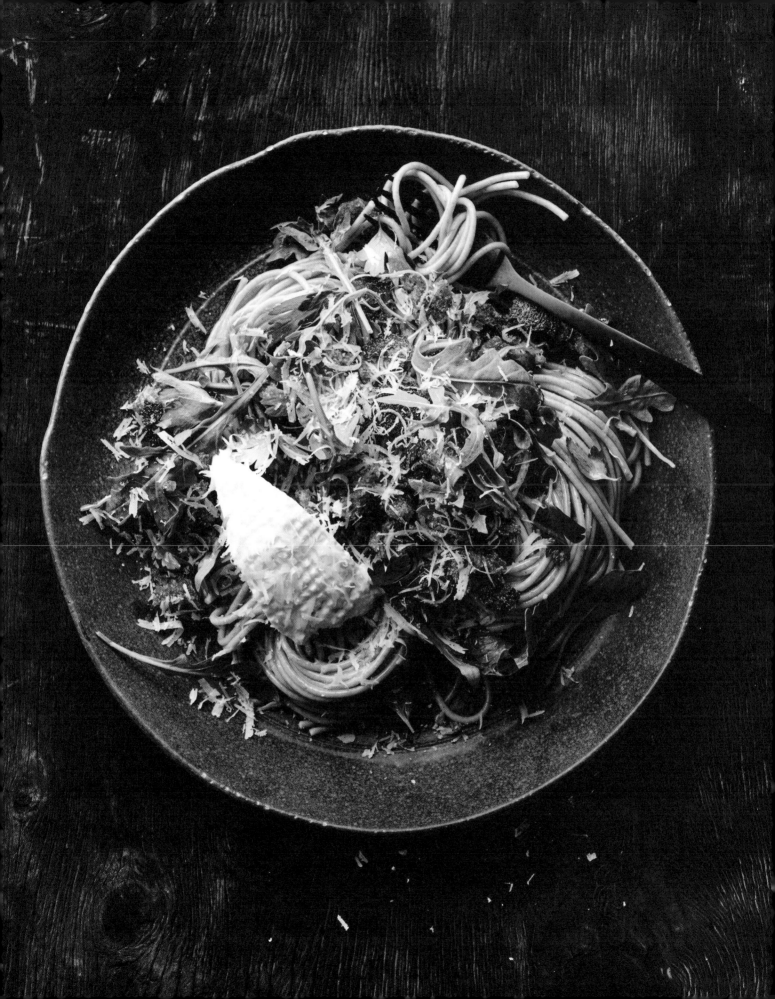

brown RICE
nasi goreng *omelette*

2 teaspoons vegetable oil
1 large red chilli, chopped
1 tablespoon finely grated ginger
2 green onions (scallions), sliced, plus extra to serve
100g (3½ oz) chicken mince
1 cup (165g/5¾ oz) cooked brown rice
1 tablespoon soy sauce
4 eggs, lightly beaten
¼ cup (60ml/2 fl oz) milk
Thai basil leaves, chilli sauce and kecap manis (sweet soy sauce),
   to serve

Heat a medium non-stick frying pan over medium heat. Add the oil,
chilli, ginger and onion and cook for 1 minute. Add the chicken mince
and cook, stirring, for 3 minutes or until just cooked through. Add the
rice and soy and cook for 1 minute.

   Whisk together the eggs and milk and add to the pan, swirling so the
egg mixture coats the bottom of the pan and distributes through the
chicken and rice mixture. Cook for 5–6 minutes or until the egg is set.

   Cut into quarters and divide among serving plates. Top with extra
green onion and basil leaves. Serve with chilli sauce and kecap manis.
SERVES 2

This recipe is the *perfect blend of two of my*
favourite STAND-BY DINNERS all made
in just one pan! *What's not to love?*

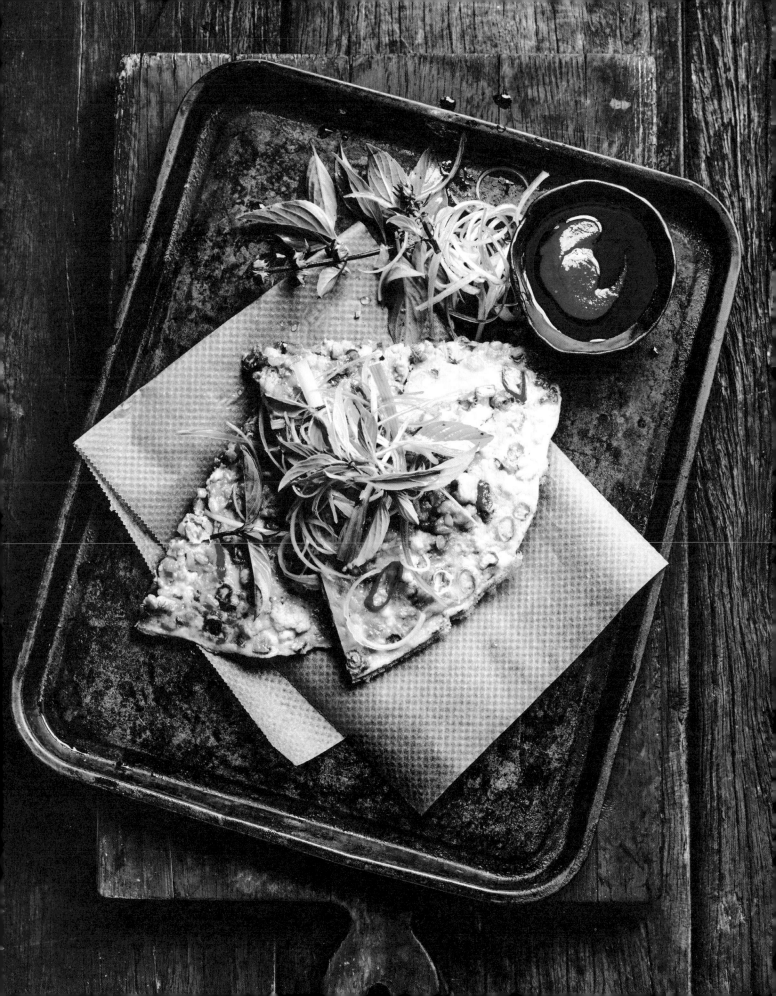

italian BAKED BEANS

2 tablespoons extra virgin olive oil
1 tablespoon salted capers, rinsed well
½ teaspoon chilli flakes
1 clove garlic, crushed
2 x 400g (14 oz) cans butter beans, drained and rinsed
2 teaspoons shredded lemon rind
2 tablespoons lemon juice
¼ cup (6g/¼ oz) flat-leaf parsley leaves
2 large slices rye or wholemeal (whole-wheat) bread, toasted
40g (1½ oz) wild rocket (arugula)
finely grated parmesan and lemon wedges (optional), to serve

Heat a large frying pan over medium heat. Add the oil and capers
and cook for 1 minute or until slightly crisp. Add the chilli and garlic
and cook for 30 seconds. Add the beans and lemon rind and cook,
stirring, for 3–4 minutes or until heated through. Stir through the
lemon juice and parsley.

Place toasts on serving plates and top with the rocket, beans and
parmesan. Serve with lemon wedges, if you like. **SERVES 2**

CREAMY butter beans are completely transformed
with *a hit of chilli, the zing of lemon and capers* and a
fresh peppery burst from the rocket. SUPER YUM!

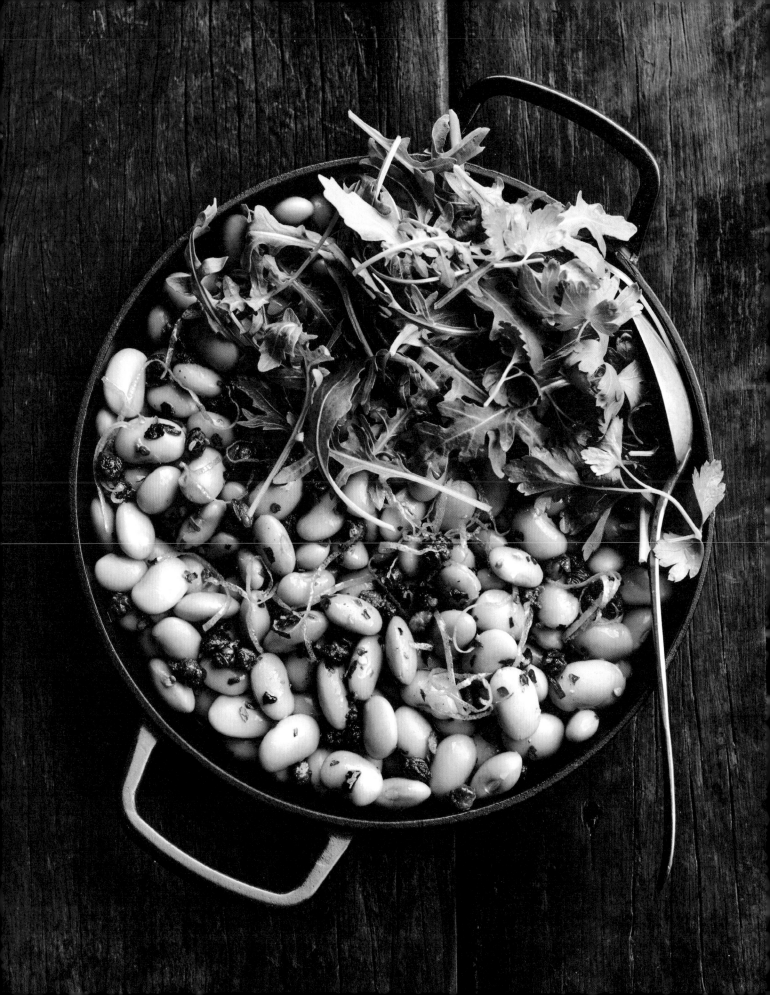

hoisin PORK dumpling *noodle soup*

4 cups (1 litre/34 fl oz) chicken stock
3 slices ginger
80g (2¾ oz) dried rice noodles
6 stalks small choy sum, trimmed and halved
2 green onions (scallions), sliced
1 green chilli, sliced
8 sprigs coriander (cilantro)
pork dumplings
200g (7 oz) pork mince[+]
2 tablespoons hoisin sauce
1 tablespoon finely grated ginger
2 tablespoons panko (Japanese) breadcrumbs
1 tablespoon chopped coriander (cilantro)

To make the pork dumplings, place the pork mince, hoisin, grated ginger, breadcrumbs and coriander in a bowl and mix well to combine.

To make the soup, place the chicken stock and sliced ginger into a saucepan over medium-low heat and simmer for 2 minutes.

Roll tablespoons of the mince mixture into balls. Add to the stock and poach for 5 minutes or until cooked through. Transfer cooked meatballs to serving bowls. Add the noodles to the stock and cook for 2 minutes or until soft. Use tongs to transfer the cooked noodles to serving bowls.

Add the choy sum to the stock and cook for 30 seconds. Divide the choy sum and stock between serving bowls. Top with green onion, chilli and coriander to serve. **SERVES 2**

+ *If you prefer, you could swap the pork mince for chicken mince.*

These are the dumplings I make when I'm *out of time to fold the dumplings in wrappers.* They're so SUPER TASTY – *all the flavour, without the fuss.*

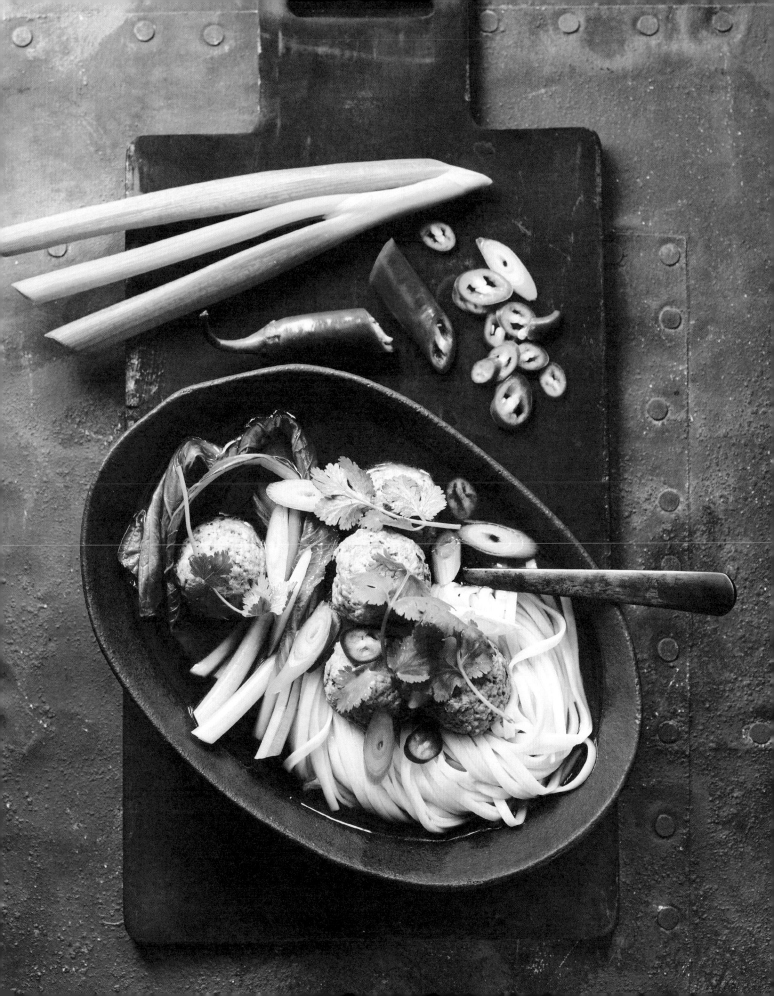

pizza WITH ARTICHOKE, mozzarella *and olives*

2 Lebanese flatbreads
⅓ cup (80ml/2¾ fl oz) tomato puree (passata)
5 artichoke hearts, halved
12 cherry tomatoes, torn and seeds removed
150g (5¼ oz) pitted green olives
2 tablespoons oregano leaves
10 thin slices fresh mozzarella, dried using paper towel
⅓ cup (25g/1 oz) finely grated parmesan
basil leaves and balsamic vinegar or thick balsamic glaze
   (optional), to serve

Preheat oven to 220°C (425°F).
   Place the flatbreads on 2 large baking trays lined with non-stick baking paper. Top each flatbread with ½ the tomato puree, artichokes, tomatoes, olives and oregano. Bake for 8 minutes.
   To serve, top each pizza with mozzarella, parmesan and basil, and drizzle with balsamic vinegar. **SERVES 2**

No need to tap for takeaway when a quick stop at THE DELI on the way home is all that's needed. *Crisp deliciousness awaits.*

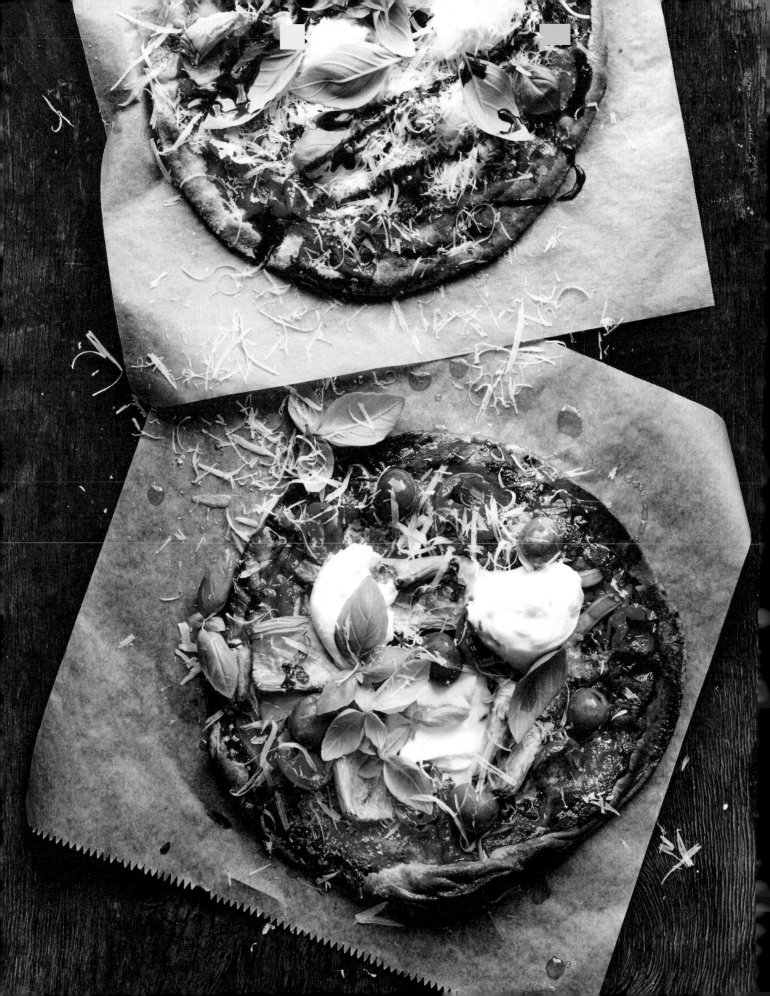

Warm LENTIL SALAD WITH lemon yoghurt *and smoked salmon*

1 tablespoon extra virgin olive oil
1 red onion, sliced
1 x 400g (14 oz) can lentils, drained
2 cups (60g/2 oz) shredded kale leaves (stems removed)
1 tablespoon red wine vinegar
sea salt and cracked black pepper
1 teaspoon finely grated lemon rind
½ cup (140g/5 oz) plain Greek-style (thick) yoghurt
6 slices smoked salmon or gravlax
lemon wedges (optional), to serve

Heat a large frying pan over medium-high heat. Add the oil and onion
and cook for 3 minutes or until soft. Add the lentils and kale and cook
for 3 minutes or until the kale is wilted and the lentils are warmed
through. Stir through the vinegar and season with salt and pepper.
Spoon onto serving plates.

Mix the lemon rind through the yoghurt and spoon onto the lentils.
Top with the smoked salmon and serve with lemon wedges if you like.

SERVES 2

This last-minute ONE-PAN no-fuss dinner is
seriously satisfying. It's bound to be high on your
new EASY DINNER rotation.

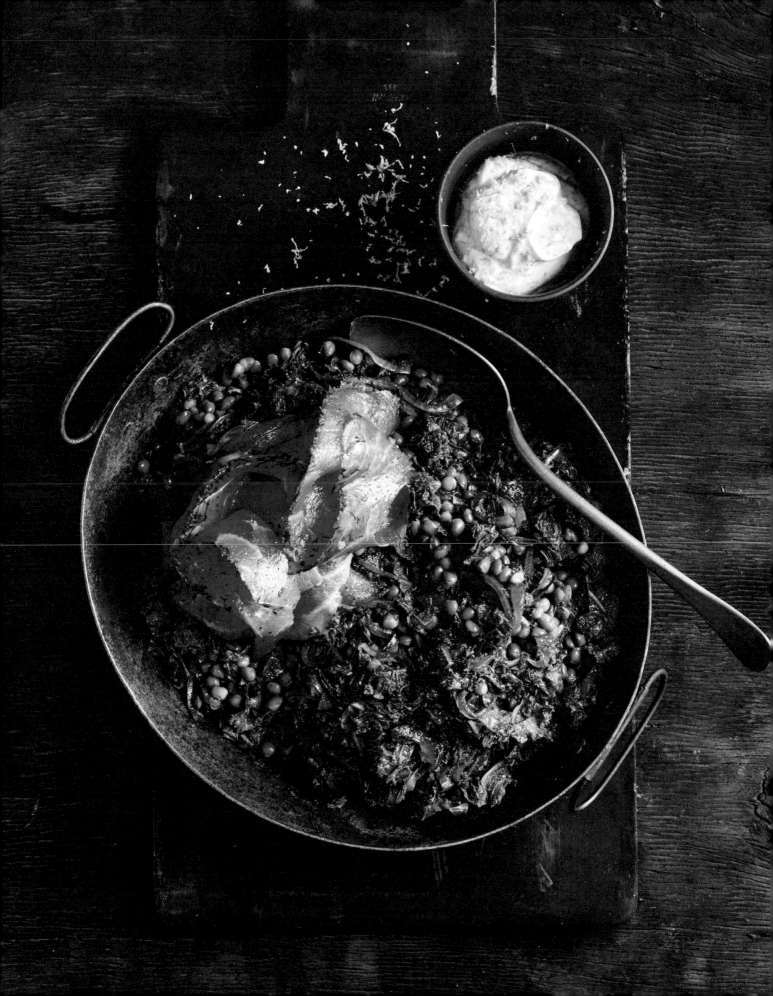

spinach SOUFFLÉ *omelette*

200g (7 oz) baby spinach leaves, blanched and finely chopped
2 tablespoons chopped dill leaves
2 tablespoons chopped flat-leaf parsley leaves
4 eggs, separated
¼ cup (60ml/2 fl oz) milk
½ cup (40g/1½ oz) finely grated parmesan, plus extra to serve
sea salt and cracked black pepper
1 tablespoon extra virgin olive oil
toasted whole-grain bread, to serve

Place the spinach, dill, parsley, egg yolks, milk, parmesan, salt and pepper in a bowl and mix to combine.

Place the egg whites into a clean bowl and whisk until soft peaks form. Fold the egg whites through the spinach mixture.

Heat a frying pan over medium heat. Add the oil and omelette mixture and cook for 4–5 minutes or until just set. Fold over and cook for a further 2 minutes.

Sprinkle with extra parmesan and serve with whole-grain toast.

SERVES 2

Enjoy a little BIT OF FANCY delicious puff *without much effort* with this super-easy one-pan omelette.

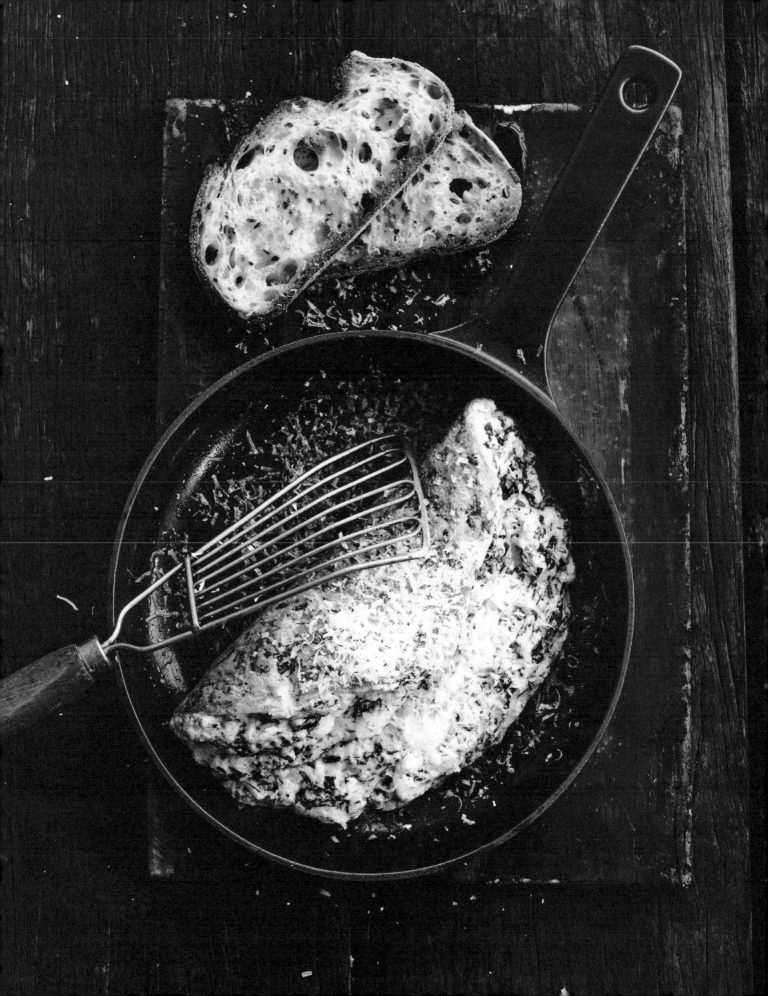

cheat's KALE, LEMON and *feta gozleme*

3 cups (90g/3 oz) shredded kale leaves (stems removed)
100g (3½ oz) baby spinach leaves
1 tablespoon grated lemon rind
150g (5¼ oz) feta, crumbled
sea salt and cracked black pepper
3 flatbreads or roti
¾ cup (180g/6¼ oz) fresh ricotta
extra virgin olive oil, for cooking
lemon cheeks, to serve

Place the kale into a bowl and cover with boiling water. Allow to stand for 2 minutes. Drain well and stir through the spinach, lemon, feta, salt and pepper.

Spread a flatbread with ⅓ of the ricotta to the edges and then place ⅓ of the kale mixture on half of the flatbread. Fold over the flatbread to enclose, making sure to press the edges firmly. Repeat with the remaining flatbreads, and the ricotta and kale mixture.

Heat a large frying pan over medium heat. Add a little oil and the flatbread and cook for 3–4 minutes each side or until golden and crisp. Cut each flatbread in half and serve with lemon cheeks. **SERVES 2**

A crispy, crunchy, much HEALTHIER and *a whole lot tastier* version of the dinner toasted sandwich. *You're welcome!*

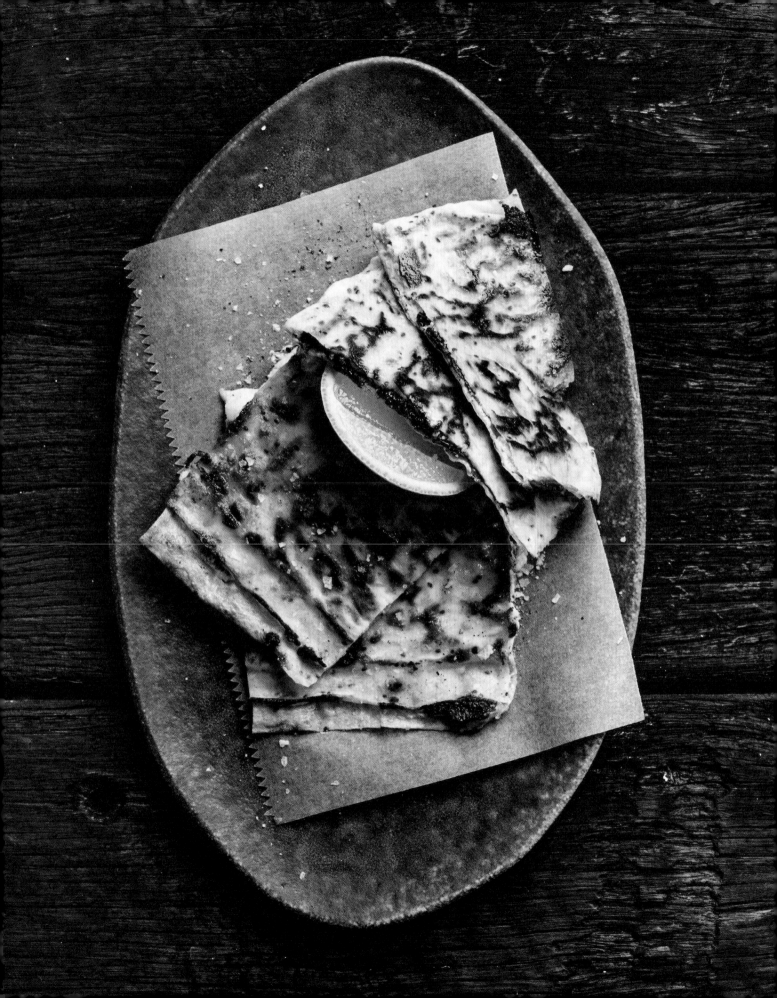

shaved SQUASH SALAD WITH smoked trout and *preserved lemon dressing*

400g (14 oz) yellow squash, thinly sliced
½ cup (8g/¼ oz) small mint leaves
¼ cup (6g/¼ oz) small dill sprigs
1 cup (20g/¾ oz) watercress sprigs
200g (7 oz) hot smoked trout fillet, broken into pieces
preserved lemon dressing
1 tablespoon shredded preserved lemon rind (pith removed),
    washed and thinly sliced
1 tablespoon honey
1½ tablespoons extra virgin olive oil
2 teaspoons lemon juice
sea salt flakes

To make the preserved lemon dressing, in a small bowl add the preserved lemon, honey, oil and lemon juice. Season with salt to taste and stir to combine.

   In a large bowl, place squash, mint, dill and watercress and drizzle with preserved lemon dressing.

   To serve, divide the shaved squash salad between bowls and top with smoked trout. **SERVES 2**

After eating these THIN AND CRISPY raw squash slices, I'll find it *hard to eat a cooked squash again.* With a zingy dressing and FRESH HERBS, *this salad is all kinds of wonderful!*

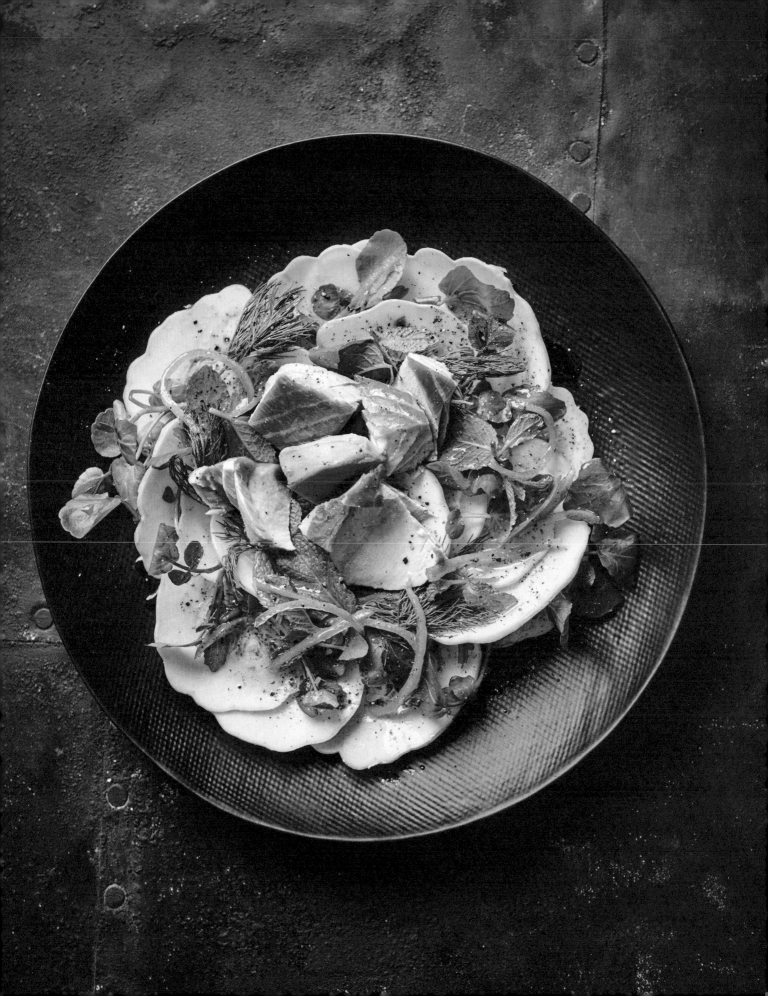

mint PESTO broccoli bowl *with blistered tomatoes*

250g (9 oz) vine-ripened cherry tomatoes
1½ tablespoons extra virgin olive oil
sea salt and cracked black pepper
100g (3½ oz) dried wholemeal (whole-wheat) spaghetti
500g (1 lb 1 oz) broccoli, about 1 large head
¼ cup (40g/1½ oz) roughly chopped almonds
1 teaspoon finely grated lemon rind
1 clove garlic, sliced
½ cup (8g/¼ oz) shredded mint leaves
1 tablespoon lemon juice
¼ cup (20g/¾ oz) finely grated parmesan, plus extra to serve
125g (4½ oz) labne, to serve

Preheat oven to 220°C (425°F).

Line a baking tray with non-stick baking paper. Place the tomatoes on the tray and drizzle with ½ the oil. Season with salt and pepper. Roast for 10 minutes or until slightly blistered.

Cook the pasta in a large saucepan of boiling salted water for 8 minutes or until al dente. Drain and set aside.

While the tomatoes and pasta are cooking, grate the broccoli on a box grater and set aside.

Heat a large non-stick frying pan over high heat. Add the remaining oil, and the almonds, lemon rind and garlic. Cook for 2 minutes or until almonds are lightly toasted. Increase heat to high, add the broccoli in 2 batches and cook, stirring, for 3 minutes or until just soft. Stir through the mint, lemon juice, parmesan, salt and pepper.

To serve, divide the pasta between bowls and top with the mint pesto broccoli, tomatoes, labne and extra grated parmesan. **SERVES 2**

This BRIGHT broccoli bowl has become our *go-to office lunch*. It's so super easy to make and still BIG on *satisfying flavours*.

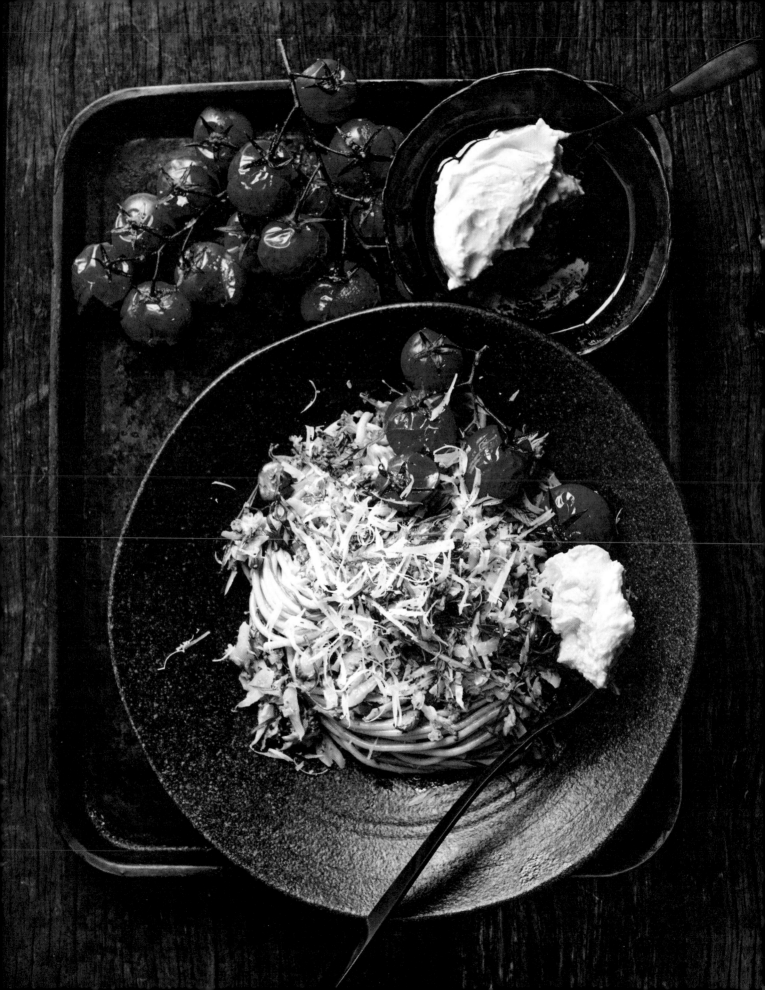

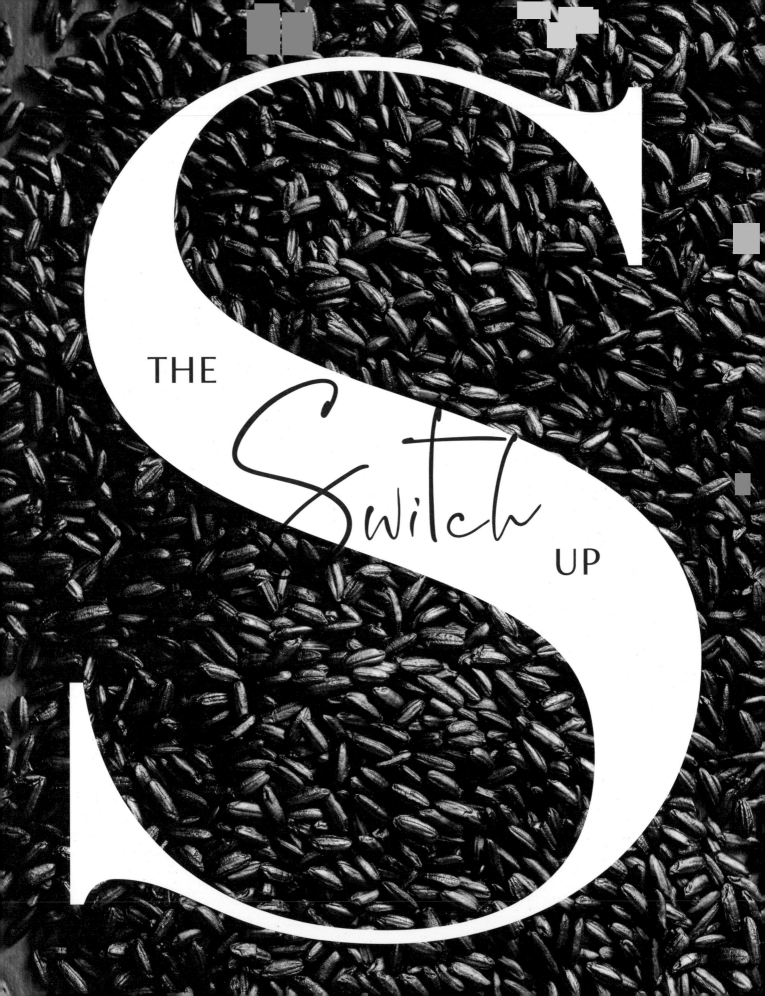

THE
Switch
UP

Almost all my recipes evolve out of my day-to-day life, but none more than the ones in this chapter. Start with a BASE FLAVOUR PROFILE or ingredient *you know your family loves*, then get creative! By simply changing-up the way you serve it or what it's paired with, you'll be rewarded with flexible meals to suit EVERY MOOD OR SEASON.

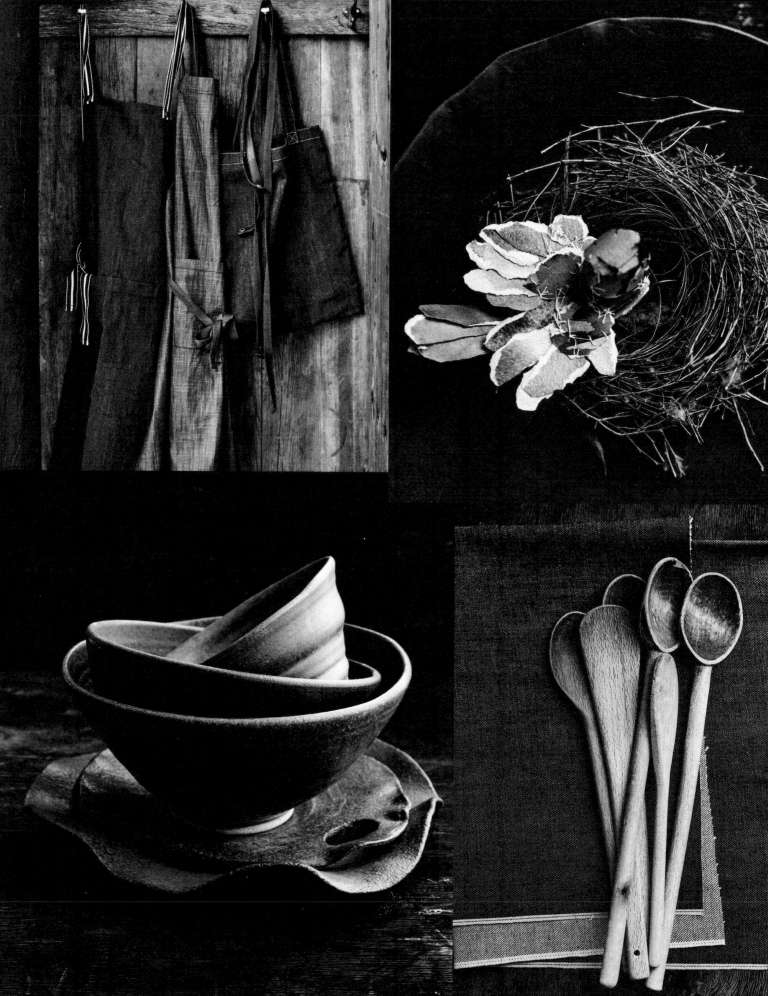

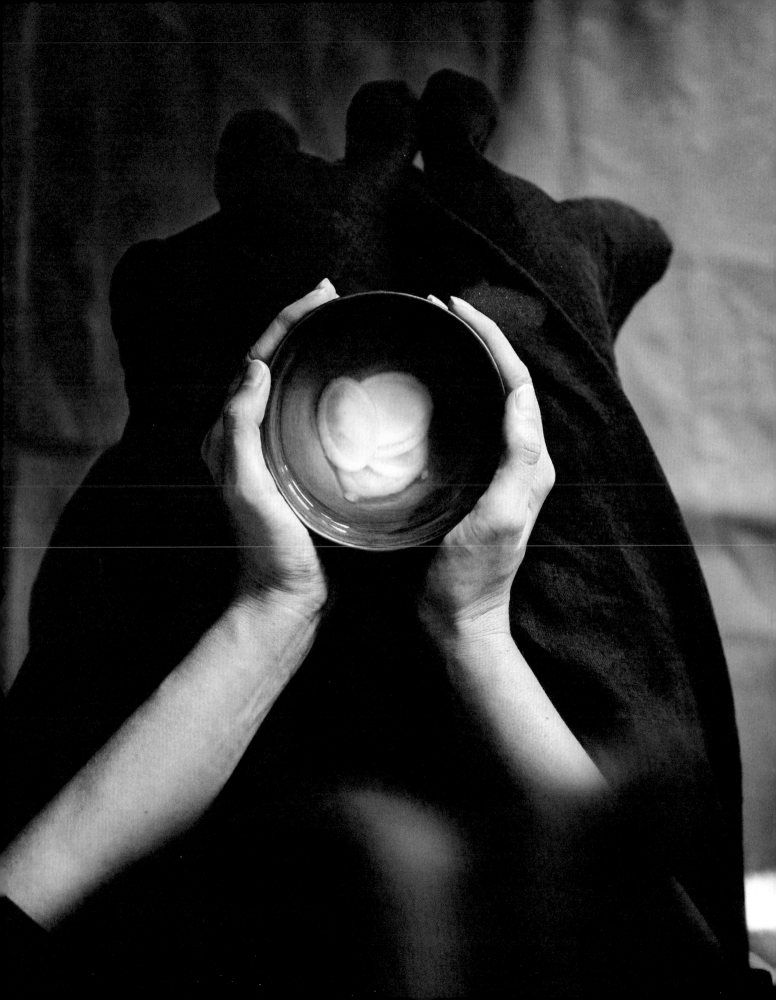

sticky MISO CHICKEN
roasted on *sesame pumpkin*

1.5kg (3lb 3 oz) butternut pumpkin (butternut squash),
   skin scrubbed and thinly sliced
2 tablespoons extra virgin olive oil
2 tablespoons sesame seeds, plus extra for sprinkling
sea salt flakes
green onion (scallion), thinly sliced and coriander (cilantro)
   leaves, to serve
sticky miso chicken
⅓ cup (95g/3¼ oz) white miso paste (shiro)
1 tablespoon sesame oil
1 tablespoon soy sauce
¼ cup (60ml/2 fl oz) mirin (Japanese rice wine)
2 tablespoons firmly packed brown sugar
1 tablespoon brown rice vinegar
6 x 125g (4½ oz) chicken thigh fillets, trimmed and halved

Preheat oven to 220°C (425°F).
   Place pumpkin, oil, sesame seeds and salt in a bowl and toss to coat.
Place on a large baking tray lined with non-stick baking paper. Roast
the pumpkin for 20 minutes.
   To make the sticky miso chicken, place the miso, oil, soy, mirin, sugar
and vinegar in a large bowl and whisk to combine. Add the chicken and
toss to coat. Set aside until ready to use.
   When the pumpkin has cooked for the 20 minutes, top the
pumpkin with the miso chicken and pour over any remaining miso
marinade. Roast for a further 20 minutes or until the chicken
is cooked through and tender.
   To serve, divide between plates, sprinkle with extra sesame
seeds and top with green onion and coriander. **SERVES 4**

The PERFECT BALANCE of salty and sweet,
miso chicken is the absolute star in these recipes.
Get creative with a SIMPLE SWITCH of veg and
herbs for a tasty new spin. *Permission granted!*

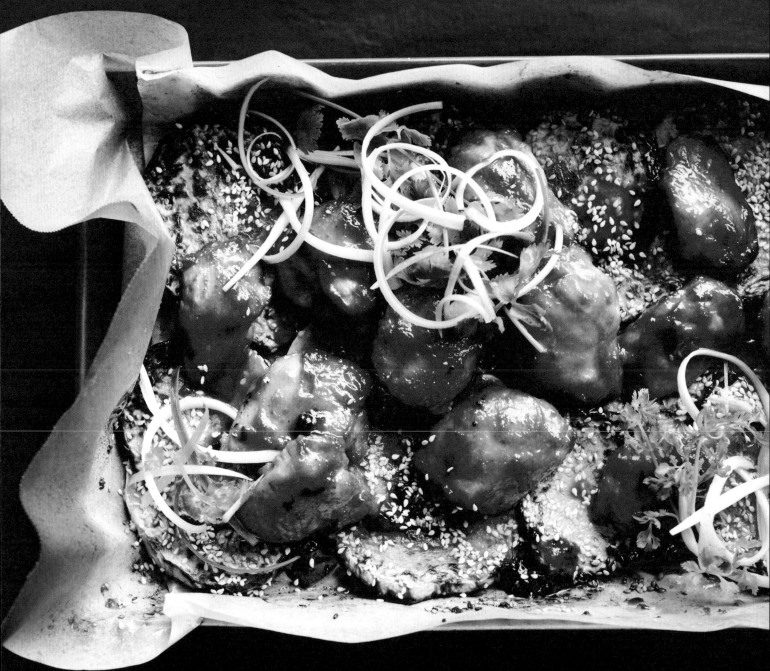

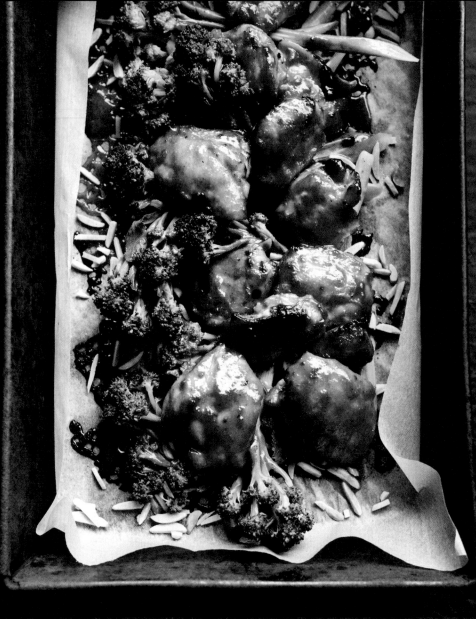

sticky MISO CHICKEN
roasted on *broccolini*

1 x quantity uncooked sticky miso chicken
  (see *recipe* p62)
4 bunches (800g/1 lb 11 oz) broccolini, trimmed
¼ cup (60ml/2 fl oz) mirin (Japanese rice wine)
2 tablespoons honey
1 tablespoon soy sauce
2 tablespoons slivered almonds

Preheat oven to 220°C (425°F).

Marinate the sticky miso chicken until ready to use.

Place the broccolini on a large baking tray lined with non-stick baking paper. In a bowl, combine mirin, honey, soy sauce and almonds. Drizzle over broccolini, top with miso chicken and any remaining marinade.

Bake for 20 minutes or until the chicken is cooked through and tender.

To serve, divide between plates. **SERVES 4**

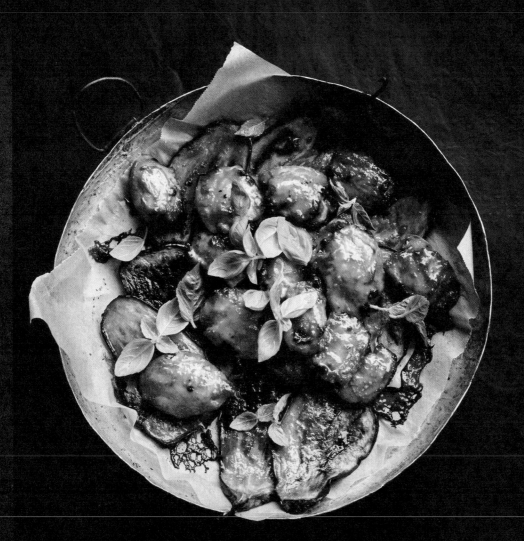

sticky MISO CHICKEN
roasted on *soy eggplant*

2 x 350g (12¼ oz) medium eggplants (aubergines), thinly sliced
1 tablespoon sesame oil
2 tablespoons soy sauce
1 tablespoon honey
1 x quantity uncooked sticky miso chicken (see *recipe* p62)
basil leaves, to serve

Preheat oven to 220°C (425°F).

Place the eggplant on a large baking tray lined with non-stick baking paper. In a bowl, combine sesame oil, soy sauce and honey. Drizzle over eggplant and roast for 20 minutes.

While the eggplant is cooking, marinate miso chicken.

When eggplant has cooked for the 20 minutes, top the eggplant with the miso chicken and any remaining marinade. Cook for a further 20 minutes or until the chicken is cooked through and tender.

Serve topped with basil leaves. **SERVES 4**

chickpea PATTIES with green tahini *and beetroot*

4 seeded buns, halved
2 large beetroot, peeled and grated
small baby beetroot leaves or lettuce leaves, to serve
salted orange sweet potato (kumara) chips, to serve
chickpea patties
2 x 400g (14 oz) cans chickpeas (garbanzo beans),
    rinsed and drained
2 tablespoons white chia seeds
⅓ cup (90g/3 oz) 'natural' crunchy peanut butter
1 tablespoon sriracha hot chilli sauce
1½ teaspoons ground cumin
1 carrot, grated
1½ cups (45g/1½ oz) finely chopped kale
sea salt and cracked black pepper
1–2 tablespoons extra virgin olive oil
green tahini
¾ cup (210g/7½ oz) hulled tahini
½ cup (125ml/4¼ fl oz) lemon juice
⅓ cup (80ml/2¾ fl oz) water
⅓ cup (4g/¼ oz) coriander leaves
⅓ cup (5g/¼ oz) mint leaves
⅓ cup (8g/¼ oz) flat-leaf parsley leaves

To make the chickpea patties, place chickpeas, chia seeds, peanut butter, sriracha and cumin into the bowl of a food processor and pulse to combine or until just roughly chopped.

Add the carrot, kale, salt and pepper and pulse lightly to just combine, then shape the mixture into 4 large flat patties.

Heat a large non-stick frying pan over medium-high heat. Add the oil and patties and cook for 6 minutes each side or until golden and crisp.

While patties are cooking, make the green tahini. Place the tahini, lemon juice, water, coriander, mint, parsley, salt and pepper in a small food process or blender and process until smooth.

To serve, spread the buns with the green tahini and divide beetroot, sorrel and chickpea patties between bases. Sandwich with the bun tops and serve with salted sweet potato chips. **SERVES 4**

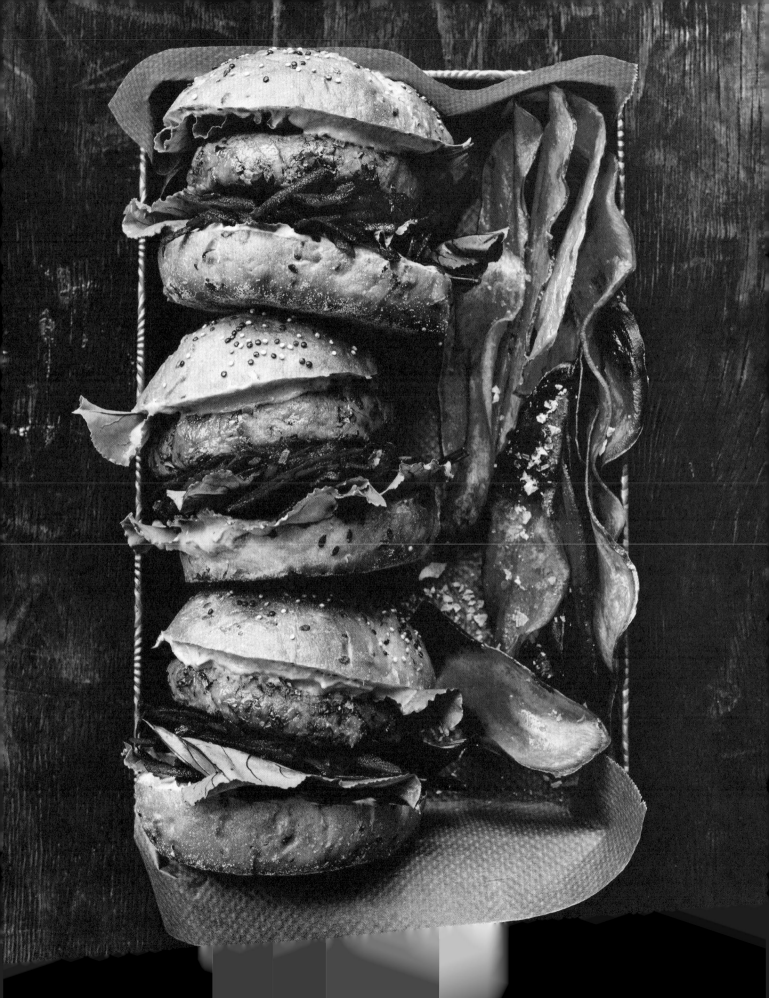

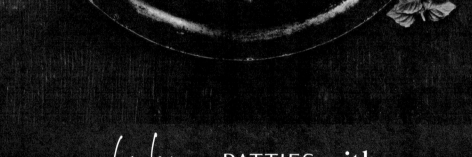

chickpea PATTIES **with**
lemon mayonnaise and parmesan pickles

radicchio, to serve
4 seeded buns, halved
1 x quantity cooked chickpea patties (see *recipe* p66)
baby shiso leaves (optional), to serve
lemon mayonnaise
⅓ cup (100g/3½ oz) whole egg mayonnaise
juice ½ lemon
parmesan pickles
6-8 pickles, halved lengthways
¼ cup (20g/½ oz) finely grated parmesan

To make the lemon mayonnaise, in a bowl add mayonnaise and lemon juice and mix to combine.

To make the parmesan pickles, press cut side of pickles into grated parmesan. Heat a non-stick frying pan over medium heat. Cook pickles parmesan-side down for 3-4 minutes or until golden.

To serve, divide radicchio between bun bases and top with chickpea patties, lemon mayonnaise and shiso leaves. Sandwich with the bun tops and serve with parmesan pickles. **SERVES 4**

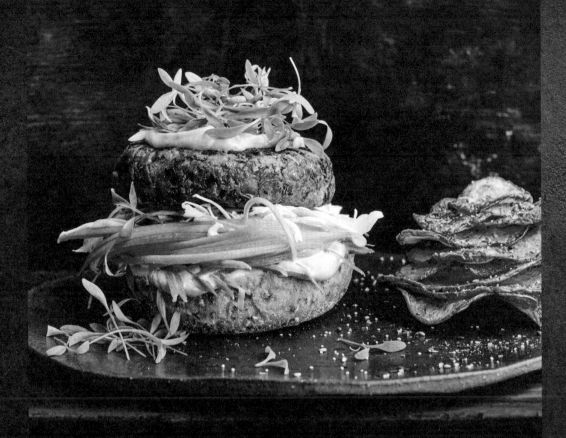

chickpea PATTIES with
miso mayonnaise and carrot slaw

4 seeded buns, halved

1 x quantity cooked chickpea patties
(see *recipe* p66)

baby coriander (cilantro) leaves, to serve

salted potato chips, to serve

carrot slaw

1 carrot, shredded using a julienne peeler

2 cups (180g/6¼ oz) thinly shaved green cabbage

2 green onions (scallions), shredded

2 teaspoons apple cider vinegar

sea salt flakes

miso mayonnaise

½ cup (150g/5¼ oz) whole egg mayonnaise

1½ teaspoons white miso paste (shiro)

To make the carrot slaw, place carrot, cabbage, onion, vinegar and salt in a bowl and toss to combine.

To make the miso mayonnaise, place mayonnaise and miso in a bowl and whisk until smooth.

To serve, spread buns with mayonnaise. Divide slaw between bun bases. Top with patties, extra mayonnaise, coriander and bun tops. Serve with chips. **SERVES 4**

free form LASAGNE
with *minted spinach*

6 fresh lasagne sheets, blanched
¼ cup (20g/¾ oz) finely grated parmesan, plus extra to serve
cauliflower cheese sauce
1kg (2 lb 3 oz) cauliflower, cut into florets
2 cups (500ml/17 fl oz) milk
¾ cup (60g/2 oz) finely grated parmesan
sea salt and cracked black pepper
minted spinach
500g (1 lb 1 oz) baby spinach leaves
¼ cup (4g/¼ oz) chopped mint leaves
¼ cup (4g/¼ oz) finely chopped chives
sea salt and cracked black pepper

Preheat oven to 220°C (425°F).
  To make the cauliflower cheese sauce, place the cauliflower
and milk in a large saucepan over low heat and bring to a simmer.
Cover with a tight-fitting lid and simmer gently for 8-10 minutes or
until the cauliflower is soft. Allow to cool slightly. Using a hand-held
stick blender, blend until smooth. Add parmesan, salt and pepper
and stir through.
  To make the minted spinach, place the spinach into a bowl and pour
over boiling water. Set aside for 30 seconds, then drain. Press the
spinach between paper towel to remove any excess liquid. Shred
the spinach and place into a bowl with the mint, chives, salt and
pepper. Mix to combine.
  To assemble lasagnes, place 1 lasagne sheet into the bases of two
lightly greased 16–18cm (6–7 inch) ovenproof dishes or frying pans. Top
each sheet with ¾-cupful of cauliflower cheese sauce, then ¼ of the
minted spinach. Repeat layering with remaining lasagne sheets,
cauliflower cheese sauce and minted spinach, finishing with the
remaining cauliflower cheese sauce. Top with the parmesan and
place dishes on a baking tray. Bake for 25 minutes or until golden
and bubbling. Serve sprinkled with the extra parmesan. **SERVES 4**

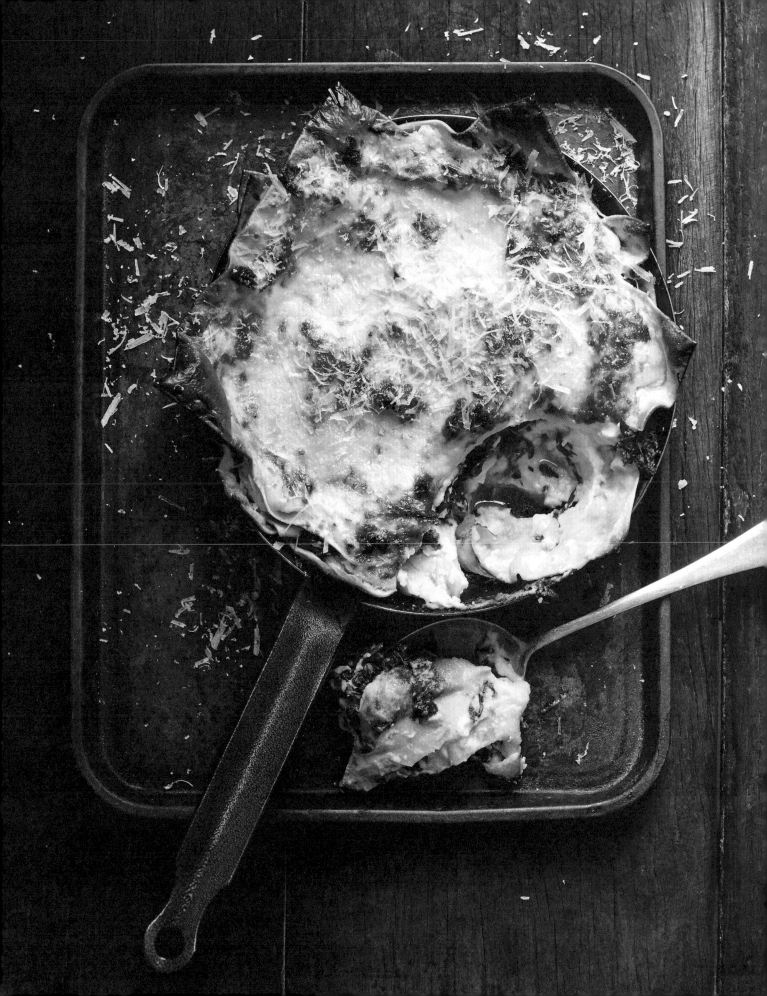

free-form LASAGNE
with *cavolo nero*

6 cups (180g/6¼ oz) shredded cavolo nero
  (Tuscan kale) (about 2 bunches), blanched
2 tablespoons chopped dill leaves
sea salt and cracked black pepper
6 fresh lasagne sheets, blanched
1 x quantity cauliflower cheese sauce
  (see *recipe* p70)
¼ cup (20g/¾ oz) finely grated parmesan
8 thin slices pancetta, halved

Preheat oven to 220°C (425°C). Place cavolo nero, dill, salt and pepper in a bowl. Mix to combine.

To assemble lasagnes, place 1 lasagne sheet into the bases of 2 lightly greased 16–18cm (6–7 inch) ovenproof dishes or frying pans. Top with ¾-cupful of cheese sauce, then ¼ of the cavolo nero mixture. Repeat layering with remaining lasagne sheets, cheese sauce and cavolo nero mixture, finishing with remaining cheese sauce. Top with parmesan and pancetta. Place on a baking tray and bake for 25 minutes or until golden and bubbling. **SERVES 4**

free-form LASAGNE
with *sage and pumpkin*

1.5kg (3lb 3 oz) pumpkin, peeled and cut into
  1cm (¼ inch) thick slices
1 tablespoon extra virgin olive oil
⅓ cup (8g/¼ oz) sage leaves, plus extra for garnish
sea salt and cracked black pepper
6 fresh lasagne sheets, blanched
1 x quantity cauliflower cheese sauce
  (see *recipe* p70)
¼ cup (20g/¾ oz) finely grated parmesan

Preheat oven to 200°C (400°F). Place pumpkin onto a large baking tray lined with non-stick baking paper. Drizzle with oil and sprinkle with sage, salt and pepper. Roast for 20 minutes, turning halfway through cooking. Increase heat to 220°C (425°F). To assemble lasagnes, place 1 lasagne sheet into bases of 2 greased 16–18cm (6–7 inch) ovenproof dishes or frying pans. Top with ¾-cupful of cheese sauce, then ¼ of pumpkin. Repeat layering with sheets, sauce and pumpkin, finishing with sauce. Top with parmesan and extra sage. Place on an oven tray. Bake for 25 minutes, until golden. **SERVES 4**

zucchini 3-CHEESE RAVIOLI
with *baked tomato sauce*

extra virgin olive oil, for brushing
basil leaves, to serve
baked tomato sauce
750g (1 lb 10 oz) cherry tomatoes
2 tablespoons extra virgin olive oil
6 small sprigs of thyme
½ cup (125ml/4½ fl oz) chicken or vegetable stock
2 tablespoons red wine vinegar
1 tablespoon pure maple syrup
sea salt and cracked black pepper
zucchini 3-cheese ravioli
1½ cups (360g/12½ oz) fresh ricotta
½ cup (40g/1½ oz) finely grated parmesan,
    plus extra to serve
150g (5 oz) soft goat's cheese
2 tablespoons chopped chives
sea salt and cracked black pepper
6 zucchini (courgettes), thinly sliced on a mandoline

Preheat oven to 200°C (400°F).

To make the baked tomato sauce, make a small cut into each tomato, squeeze out and discard seeds. Place tomatoes into a large baking dish with the oil, thyme, stock, vinegar, maple, salt and pepper and bake for 20 minutes or until soft.

To make the zucchini 3-cheese ravioli, place ricotta, parmesan, goat's cheese, chives, salt and pepper into a bowl and mix to combine. On a board, lay 4 slices of zucchini overlapping each other in the centre (it will look like a star). Place a heaped tablespoon of cheese mixture in the centre, then fold over zucchini to enclose filling. Turn over the ravioli so the zucchini ends are underneath. Repeat with remaining zucchini and cheese mixture.

Place the zucchini ravioli on top of hot tomato sauce. Brush with oil and bake for 20 minutes or until the edges of the zucchini are lightly golden. Serve scattered with a little extra parmesan and basil leaves.

SERVES 4

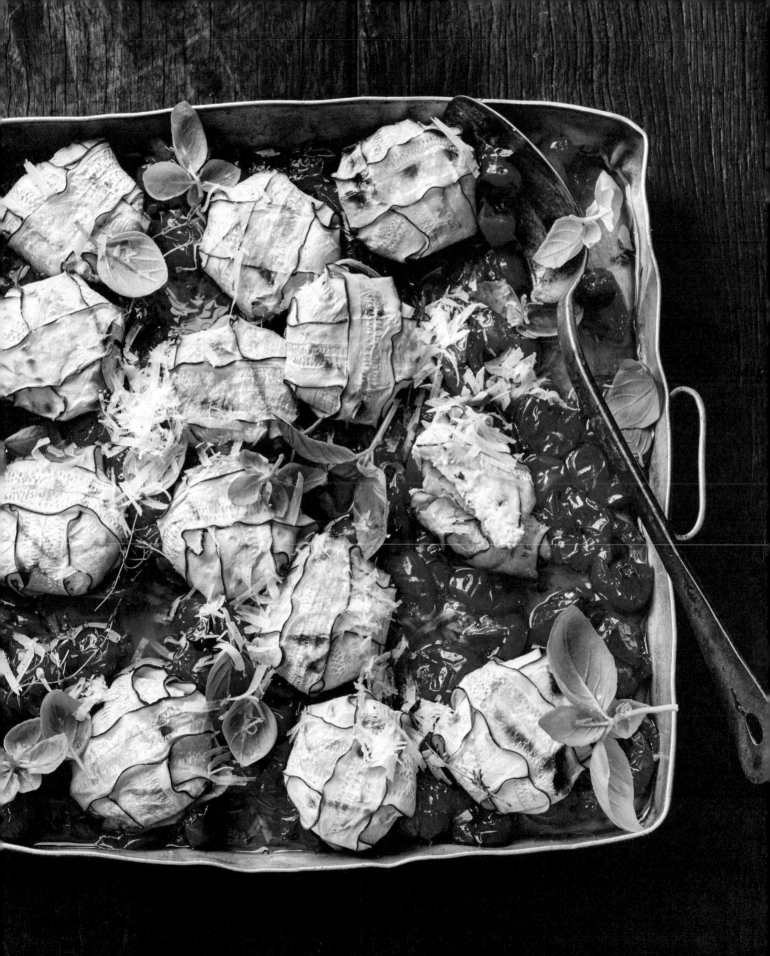

zucchini, SPINACH and *ricotta ravioli*

1 x quantity uncooked baked tomato sauce (see p74)

1⅓ cups (320g/11 oz) fresh ricotta

⅓ cup (25g/1 oz) finely grated parmesan,
  plus extra to serve

200g (7 oz) frozen spinach, defrosted (excess
  moisture removed) and chopped

2 tablespoons chopped dill

sea salt and cracked black pepper

6 zucchini (courgettes), thinly sliced on a mandoline

extra virgin olive oil, for brushing

red-veined sorrel, to serve

Preheat oven to 200°C (400°F). While baked tomato sauce is cooking, make ravioli. Combine the ricotta, parmesan, spinach, dill, salt and pepper. On a board, lay 4 slices of zucchini overlapping in centre (it will look like a star). Place a heaped tablespoon of spinach mixture in centre, then fold over zucchini to enclose filling. Turn over the ravioli so the zucchini ends are underneath. Repeat with remaining zucchini and spinach mixture. Place ravioli onto the hot tomato sauce. Brush with oil. Bake for 20 minutes, until edges of zucchini are light golden. Serve with extra parmesan and sorrel. **SERVES 4**

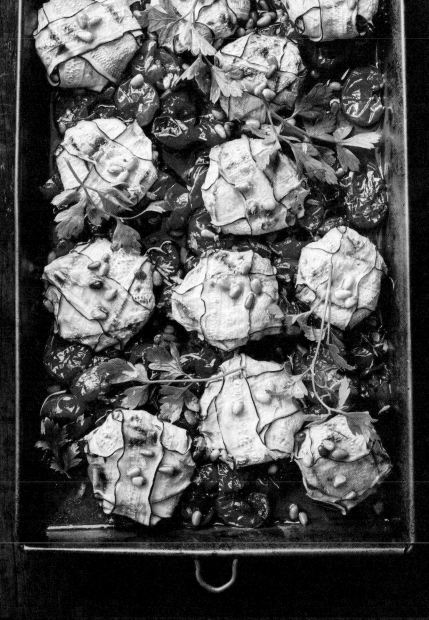

zucchini, CHICKEN, KALE and *pine nut ravioli*

1 x quantity uncooked baked tomato sauce (see p74)

1½ cups (45g/1½ oz) shredded kale leaves, blanched

150g (5 oz) chicken mince

½ cup (120g/4½ oz) fresh ricotta

2 tablespoons chopped flat-leaf parsley leaves

¼ cup (40g/1½ oz) toasted pine nuts,
  plus extra to serve

1 tablespoon finely grated lemon rind

sea salt and cracked black pepper

6 zucchini (courgettes), thinly sliced on a mandoline

extra virgin olive oil, for brushing

Preheat oven to 200°C (400°F). While baked tomato sauce is cooking, make ravioli. Combine the kale, chicken, ricotta, parsley, nuts, zest, salt and pepper. On a board, lay 4 slices of zucchini overlapping in centre (it will look like a star). Place a heaped tablespoon of chicken mixture in centre. Fold over zucchini to enclose filling. Turn over the ravioli so the zucchini ends are underneath. Repeat with zucchini and chicken mixture. Place ravioli onto hot tomato sauce. Brush with oil. Bake for 20 minutes, until zucchini is light golden. Serve with extra nuts and parsley. **SERVES 4**

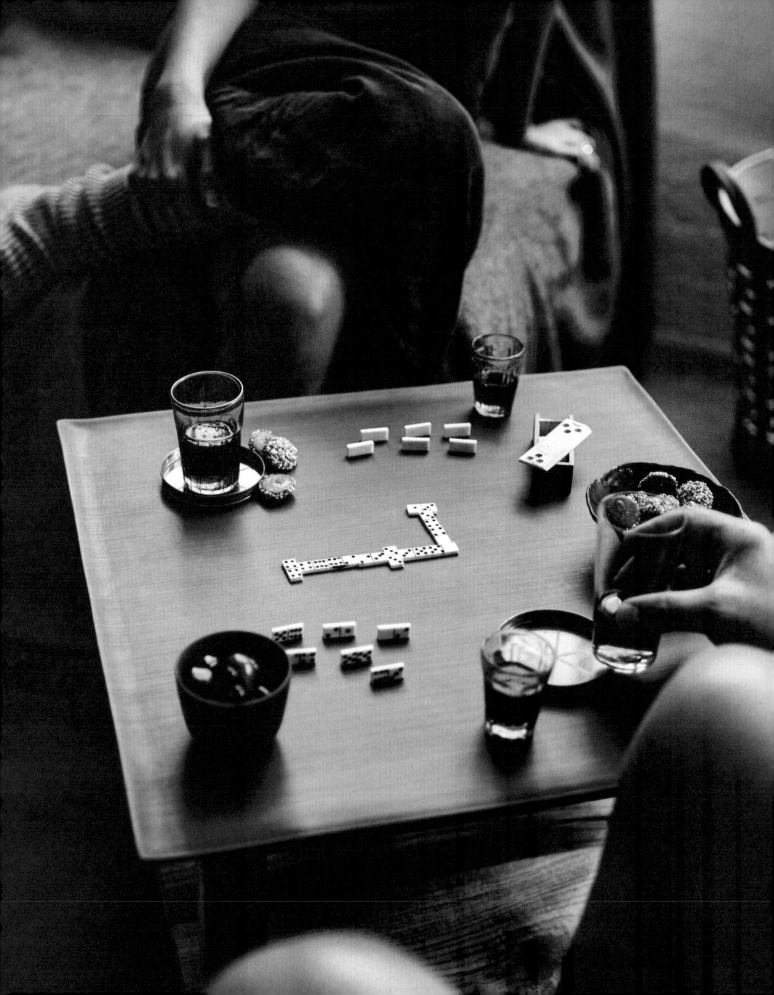

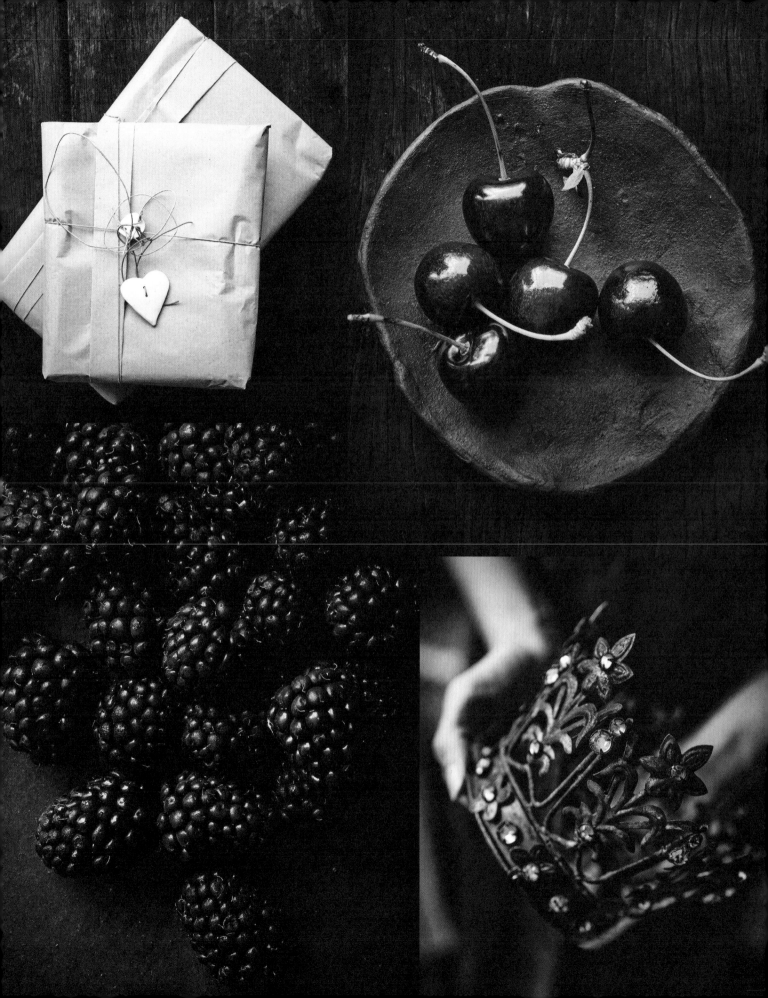

cauliflower RICE BOWLS
with *crispy chilli eggs*

cauliflower rice bowls
2 tablespoons extra virgin olive oil
2 cloves garlic, sliced
2 tablespoons oregano leaves
1kg (2 lb 3 oz) cauliflower, grated
sea salt and cracked black pepper
200g (7 oz) baby spinach leaves
crispy chilli eggs
1 tablespoon extra virgin olive oil
2 large red chillies, chopped
1 green onion (scallion), chopped
4 eggs

To make the cauliflower rice bowls, heat a large frying pan over high heat. Add the oil, garlic and oregano and cook for 1 minute. Add the cauliflower, salt and pepper and cook, stirring, for 5 minutes or until cauliflower is soft. Stir through baby spinach.

To make the crispy chilli eggs, heat a medium frying pan over high heat. Add the oil, chilli and onion and cook for 1 minute. Break the eggs into the pan and cook for 1 minute. Reduce temperature to low and cover pan. Cook for 2 minutes or until the eggs are cooked to your liking.

To serve, place the cauliflower rice mixture into bowls and top with a chilli egg. **SERVES 4**

My favourite NEW WAY to make cauliflower rice is to *simply grate it on a trusty box grater.* No need to drag out the food processor every time. It's one of those things I wish I'd discovered sooner. SO EASY *that I now make it much more often.*

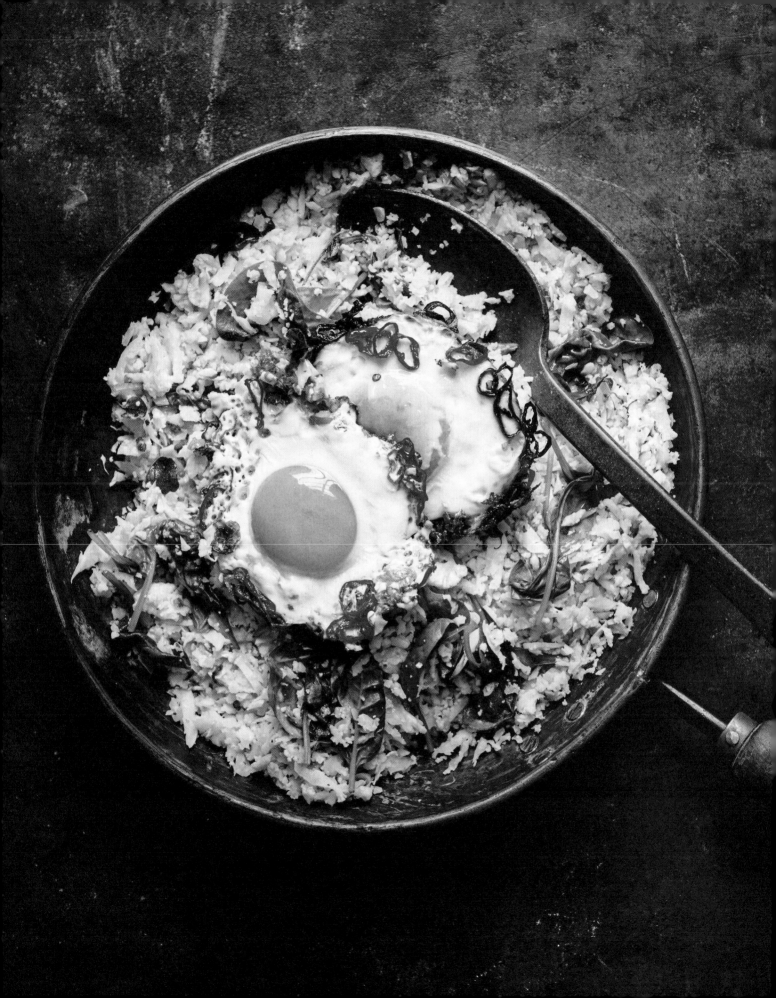

cauliflower RICE BOWLS with *chilli black beans and toasted corn*

1 x quantity cooked cauliflower rice bowls (see p80)
1 avocado, quartered, to serve
coriander (cilantro) leaves and lime cheeks and
  charred large green chilli, to serve
chilli black beans and toasted corn
1 tablespoon extra virgin olive oil
2 corncobs, kernels removed
2 large green chillies, sliced
2 teaspoons smoked paprika
400g (14 oz) can black beans, drained and rinsed
200g (7 oz) cherry tomatoes, quartered

To make the chilli black beans and toasted corn, heat a medium frying pan over high heat. Add the oil and corn and cook for 4 minutes. Add the chilli and paprika and cook for 5 minutes or until the corn has slightly blackened edges. Remove from heat and stir through the black beans and cherry tomatoes.

To serve, divide cooked cauliflower rice between bowls and top with the chilli black beans and toasted corn, the avocado, coriander, lime cheeks and charred chilli. **SERVES 4**

cauliflower RICE BOWLS **with**
smoked trout and cucumber yoghurt

1 x quantity cooked cauliflower rice bowls
** (see *recipe* p80)**
320g (11 oz) hot smoked trout fillet, roughly flaked
rocket (arugula) and extra mint leaves, to serve
cucumber yoghurt
1 x 125g (4½ oz) Lebanese cucumber, finely chopped
1 cup (245g/8¾ oz) plain Greek-style (thick) yoghurt
1 teaspoon finely grated lemon rind
½ cup (8g/¼ oz) shredded mint leaves
¼ cup (35g/1¼ oz) chopped cornichons
sea salt and cracked black pepper

To make the cucumber yoghurt, place the cucumber, yoghurt, lemon rind, mint, cornichons, salt and pepper in a bowl and mix to combine.

To serve, divide the cooked cauliflower rice between bowls and top with cucumber yoghurt, trout, rocket and extra mint leaves. **SERVES 4**

ricotta FRITTATAS with *herbed kale and roasted tomatoes*

8 vine-ripened cherry tomatoes
1 tablespoon extra virgin olive oil
sea salt and cracked black pepper
½ cup (12g/½ oz) flat-leaf parsley leaves
3 cups (90g/3 oz) finely shredded kale leaves (stems removed)
½ cup (40g/1½ oz) finely grated parmesan
½ cup (10g/¼ oz) basil leaves
ricotta frittata mixture
6 eggs
¼ cup (60ml/2 fl oz) milk
1 cup (240g/8½ oz) fresh ricotta
sea salt and cracked black pepper

Preheat oven to 200°C (400°F).

Line an 8-hole ½-cup-capacity muffin tin with deep muffin papers.

Place the tomatoes on a large baking tray lined with non-stick baking paper. Drizzle tomatoes with oil, sprinkle with salt and pepper and roast for 20 minutes or until slightly blistered.

While the tomatoes are cooking, make the ricotta frittata mixture. Place the eggs, milk, ricotta, salt and pepper in a bowl and mix to combine.

Fill a large bowl with iced water. In a separate large bowl, place the parsley and kale and pour over boiling water. Blanch for 20 seconds, then immediately drain and transfer to the iced water to refresh, before draining.

Add kale mixture to the ricotta frittata mixture, along with the parmesan and basil. Fold through.

Reduce oven temperature to 180°C (350°F). Divide frittata mixture between muffin cases, top with a tomato and bake for 20-25 minutes or until golden. **SERVES 4**

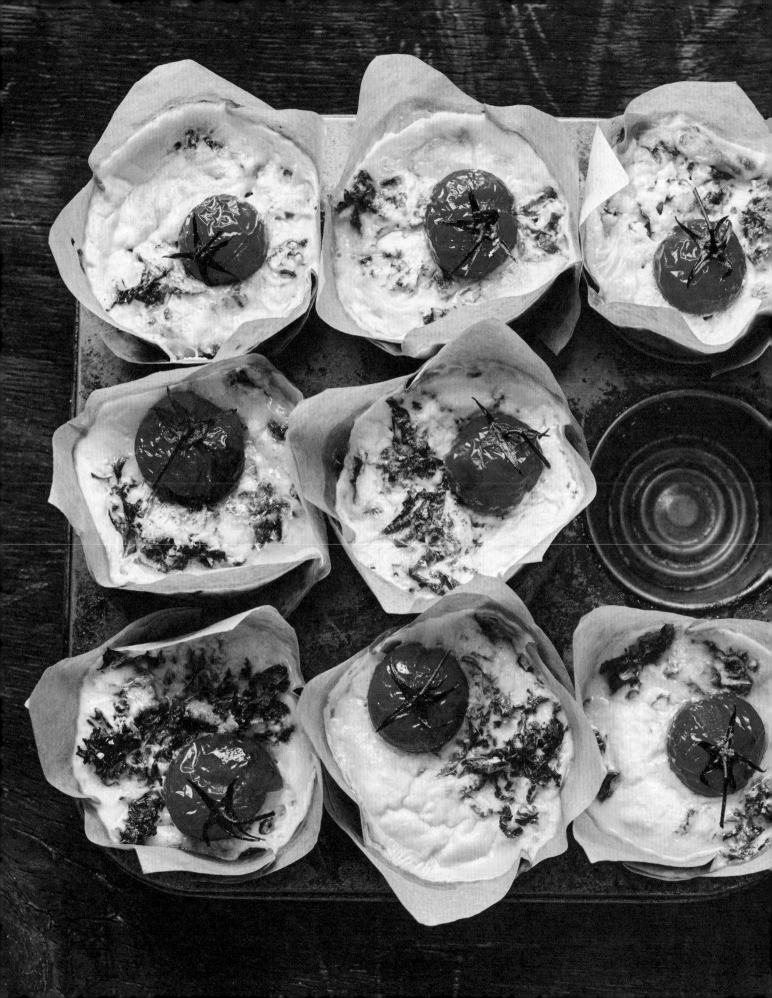

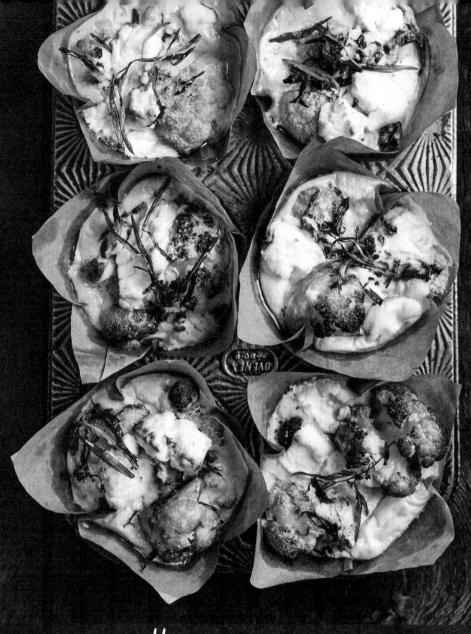

ricotta FRITTATAS with
tarragon roasted cauliflower

1kg (2 lb 3 oz) cauliflower florets

¼ cup (12g/½ oz) tarragon leaves, reserving
1 tablespoon to garnish

2 tablespoons extra virgin olive oil

100g (3½ oz) soft goat's cheese

1 x quantity uncooked ricotta frittata mixture
(see *recipe* p84)

Preheat oven to 200°C (400°F). Line an 8-hole ½-cup-capacity muffin tin with deep muffin papers. Place cauliflower, tarragon and oil into a large bowl and toss to combine.

Place cauliflower and tarragon on a large baking tray lined with non-stick baking paper. Roast for 25 minutes or until golden. Reduce oven to 180°C (350°F). Divide cauliflower mixture between muffin cases. Crumble over the cheese. Divide the ricotta frittata mix between muffin cases and scatter with reserved tarragon. Bake for 20-25 minutes or until golden. **SERVES 4**

ricotta FRITTATAS
with *minted peas and feta*

2 cups (240g/8½ oz) fresh peas, blanched
  and roughly smashed
2 tablespoons finely chopped chives
¼ cup (4g/¼ oz) mint leaves
100g (3½ oz) feta, crumbled
1 tablespoon extra virgin olive oil
sea salt and cracked black pepper
1 x quantity uncooked ricotta frittata mixture
  (see *recipe* p84)

Preheat oven to 180°C (350°F). Line an 8-hole
½-cup-capacity muffin tin with deep muffin papers.
  Place the peas, chives, mint, feta, oil, salt and pepper
into a bowl and stir to combine.
  Divide the minted pea mixture between muffin cases
and top with the ricotta frittata mixture. Bake for
20-25 minutes or until golden. **SERVES 4**

cauliflower PIZZA with tomato, *prosciutto and rocket*

24 vine-ripened cherry tomatoes
extra virgin olive oil, to cook
sea salt and cracked black pepper
100g (3½ oz) thinly sliced prosciutto, to serve
baby rocket (arugula) leaves, finely grated parmesan and
  vincotto or balsamic glaze, to serve
cauliflower pizza bases
1 cup (160g/5½ oz) pepitas (pumpkin seeds)
600g (1 lb 3 oz) cauliflower florets, roughly chopped
2 tablespoons nutritional yeast (optional)
3 eggs, lightly whisked
½ cup (40g/1½ oz) finely grated parmesan
sea salt and cracked black pepper

Preheat oven to 200°C (400°F).
  To make the cauliflower pizza bases, place the pepitas into the
bowl of a food processor and process until finely ground. Add the
cauliflower, yeast, eggs, parmesan, salt and pepper. Process until
very finely chopped and dough like.
  Press the mixture onto 2 x 28cm (11 inch) round pizza trays lined
with non-stick baking paper. Bake for 20 minutes or until golden.
  Place the tomatoes on a large baking tray lined with non-stick
baking paper. Drizzle tomatoes with oil and sprinkle with salt and
pepper. Roast for 20 minutes or until golden.
  To serve, top the bases with tomatoes, prosciutto, rocket,
and parmesan. Finish with a drizzle of vincotto or balsamic glaze.
SERVES 4

This is an updated, UPFLAVOURED version of
my favourite cauliflower pizza base. I love the nutty
taste pepitas bring to this while still keeping
it NUT FREE. If you can get your hands on
nutritional yeast, it's absolutely worth it for the
savoury depth of flavour it brings to the pizza.

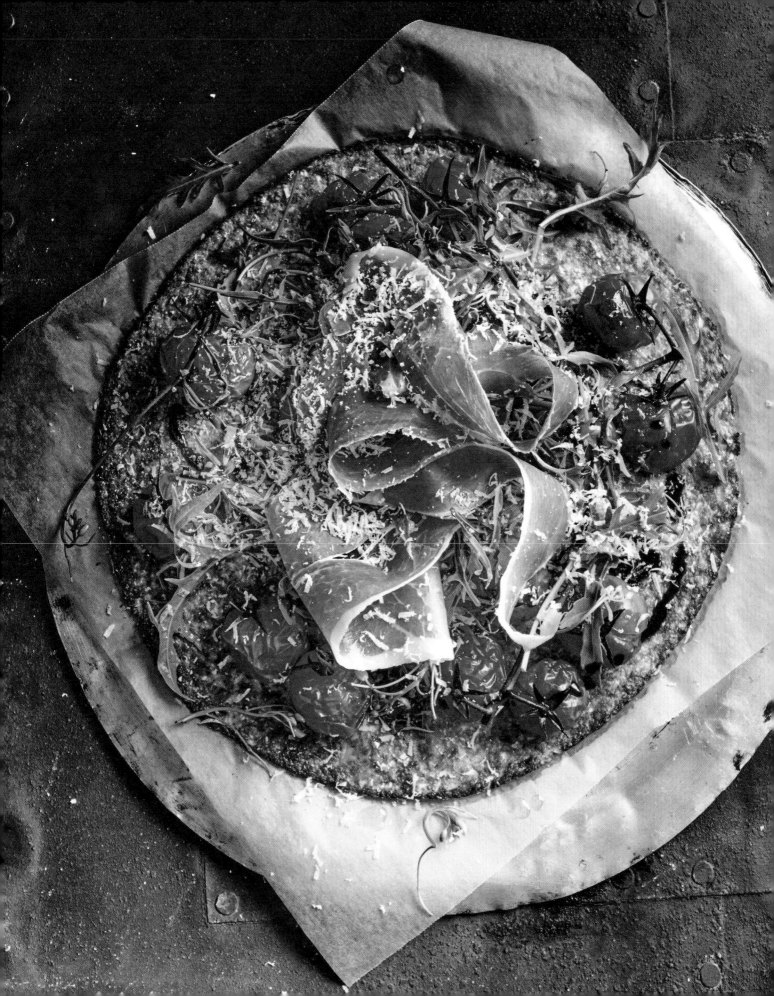

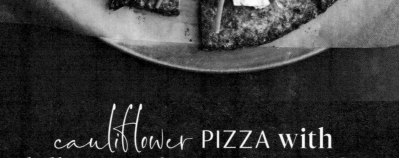

cauliflower PIZZA with
chilli-roasted pumpkin and feta

800g (1 lb 7 oz) pumpkin, thinly sliced

1 red onion, cut into wedges

1 tablespoon extra virgin olive oil, plus extra to drizzle

¼ teaspoon chilli flakes, plus extra to serve

1 x quantity cooked cauliflower pizza bases (see
  recipe p88)

150g (5 oz) feta

½ cup (12g/½ oz) baby spinach leaves

Preheat oven to 200°C (400°F).

Place pumpkin and onion on a large baking tray lined with non-stick baking paper. Drizzle with oil and sprinkle with chilli. Roast for 20 minutes.

To serve, top each warm cauliflower pizza base with the roasted pumpkin and onion. Crumble over the feta and scatter with spinach. Serve with a drizzle of oil and extra chilli. **SERVES 4**

cauliflower PIZZA with
beetroot and goat's cheese

1 x quantity cooked cauliflower pizza bases
   (see *recipe* p88)

6 target or baby beetroot, scrubbed and
   thinly sliced using a mandoline, small
   leaves reserved

150g (5 oz) soft goat's cheese

extra virgin olive oil and pomegranate molasses or
   balsamic glaze, to serve

Top each warm cauliflower pizza base with the
beetroot slices and beetroot leaves and crumble over
the goat's cheese.

Serve with a drizzle of oil and pomegranate molasses

SERVES 4

maple TERIYAKI SALMON
with *lettuce cups and pickles*

8 cos (romaine) lettuce leaves
2 cups (330g/11½ oz) cooked jasmine rice
2 green onions (scallions), thinly sliced on the diagonal
mint leaves, coriander (cilantro) leaves and lime wedges, to serve
maple teriyaki salmon
¼ cup (60ml/2 fl oz) pure maple syrup
¼ cup (60ml/2 fl oz) soy sauce
1 tablespoon finely grated ginger
1 clove garlic, finely sliced
4 x 150g (5¼ oz) skinless salmon fillets, pin boned
quick pickles
⅓ cup (80ml/2¾ fl oz) apple cider vinegar
1 tablespoon pure maple syrup
sea salt flakes
4 baby cucumbers, thinly sliced

Preheat oven to 200°C (400°F).
 For maple teriyaki salmon, in a small saucepan, add maple, soy, ginger and garlic. Simmer over medium heat for 2 minutes. Place salmon on a baking tray lined with non-stick baking paper. Spoon over maple teriyaki sauce and bake in oven for 5 minutes, basting halfway through cooking.
 For quick pickles, combine vinegar, maple and salt in a bowl. Stir through cucumber and set aside for 5 minutes.
 Fill lettuce cups with rice and maple teriyaki salmon. Serve with quick pickles, green onion, herbs and lime wedges. **SERVES 4**

The PUNCHY FLAVOURS of maple and teriyaki are best matched with a firm, *robust-flavoured fish like salmon*. Ocean trout and kingfish stand up well too. But as always, feel free to try it with whatever is FRESH, SUSTAINABLE and *local to you.*

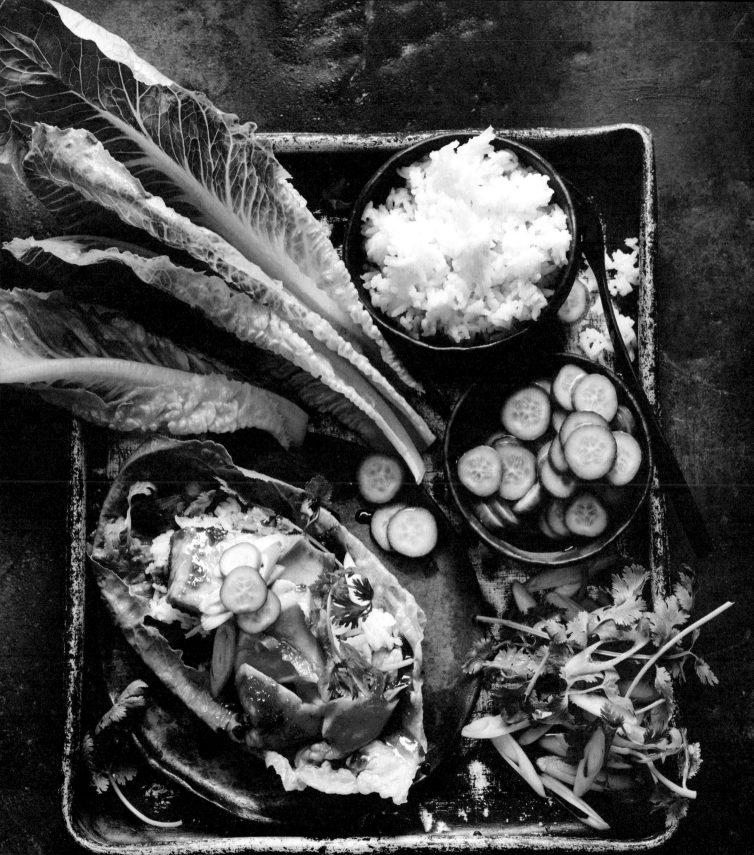

maple TERIYAKI SALMON
with *soba noodle salad*

160g (5½ oz) dried soba noodles, cooked

200g (7 oz) snow peas (mange tout), blanched

200g (7 oz) sugar snap peas, blanched and halved

100g (3½ oz) bean sprouts, tails picked

1 x quantity cooked maple teriyaki salmon (reserving
  2 tablespoons of the maple teriyaki marinade)
  (see *recipe* p92)

Divide noodles, snow peas, sugar snaps, bean sprouts and reserved teriyaki marinade between bowls.

To serve, top with the maple teriyaki salmon. **SERVES 4**

maple TERIYAKI SALMON
with *toasted nori and kale slaw*

4 nori sheets, toasted

1 x quantity cooked maple teriyaki salmon (see p92)

kale slaw

¼ cup (60ml/2 fl oz) brown rice vinegar

1 tablespoon firmly packed brown sugar

sea salt flakes

3½ cups (105g/3¾ oz) shredded kale leaves
  (stems removed)

2 carrots, shredded using a julienne peeler

2 target or small beetroot, scrubbed and thinly sliced

2 tablespoons toasted sesame seeds

To make the kale slaw, in a large bowl, add vinegar, sugar and salt and mix to combine. Add kale and rub in dressing for 2 minutes or until softened. Fold through the carrot, beetroot and sesame seeds.

To serve, divide nori between plates and top with kale slaw and maple teriyaki salmon. **SERVES 4**

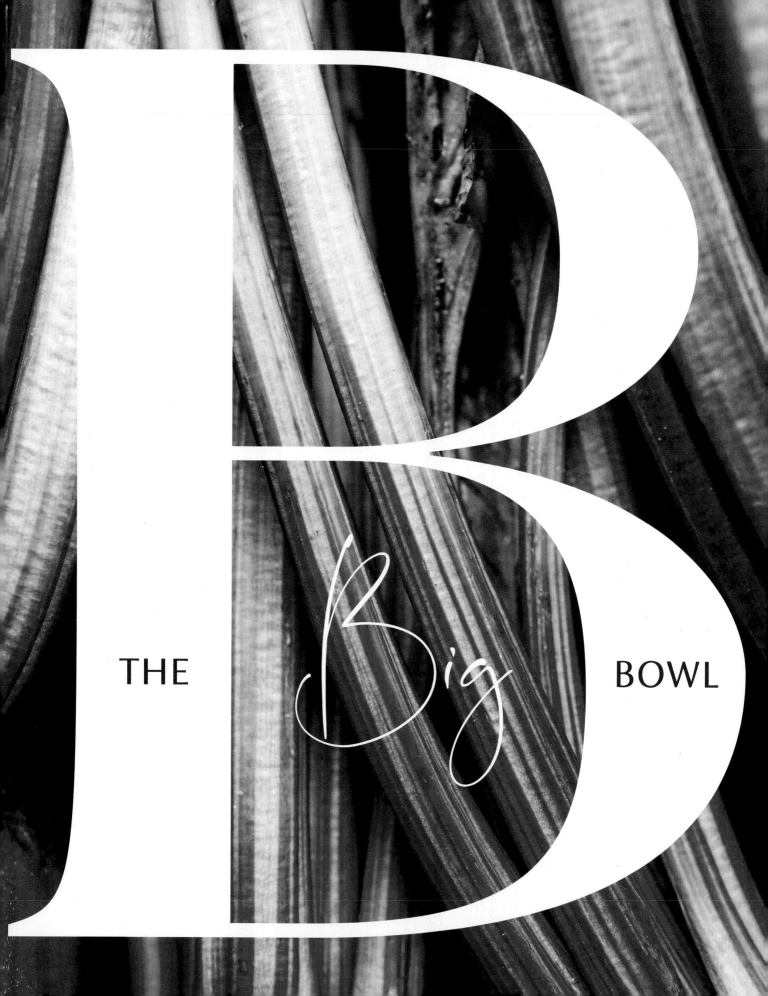

THE **B**ig BOWL

Is it me, or does everything taste better in a bowl? Vibrant, fresh and filled to the brim with fabulous flavours and textures – THE BOWL IS COMPLETE. *Vegetables feature large in these big bowls*, whether raw, pickled, roasted or grilled. Here you'll find everything you need, deliciously nestled in ONE PERFECT VESSEL.

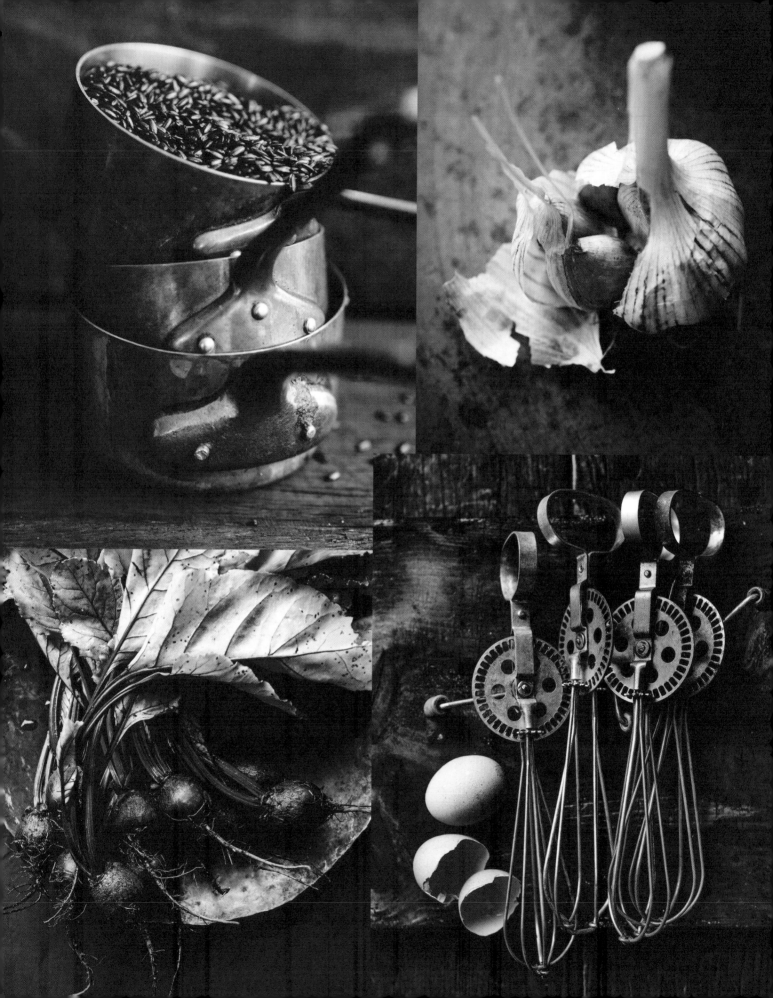

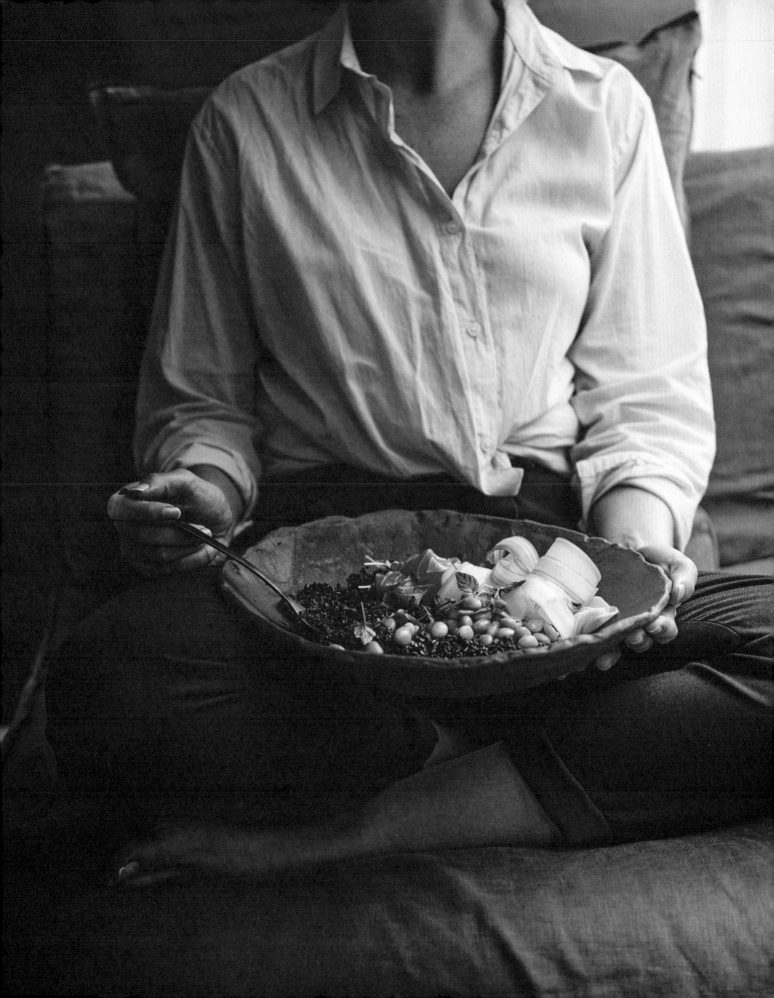

black RICE BOWL with ginger and *turmeric seared chicken*

4 cups (800g/1 lb 8 oz) cooked black rice
1 cup (140g/4¼ oz) frozen shelled edamame beans, blanched
2 small cucumbers, thinly sliced
12 small red radishes with leaves attached, halved
½ bunch coriander (cilantro), sprigs picked
turmeric chicken
1 tablespoon finely grated ginger
½ teaspoon ground turmeric
2 teaspoons extra virgin olive oil
sea salt flakes
3 x 150g (4¼ oz) small chicken breast fillets, trimmed
turmeric dressing
1 cup (280g/10 oz) plain Greek-style (thick) yoghurt
3 teaspoons finely grated ginger
1 teaspoon ground turmeric
½ teaspoon sea salt flakes

To make the turmeric chicken, place the ginger, turmeric, oil, salt and chicken together in a bowl and toss well to coat.

Heat a medium non-stick frying pan over medium heat. Cook chicken for 5 minutes on each side or until golden and cooked through. Set aside to rest for 5 minutes, then slice each breast into 4 thick slices.

To make the turmeric dressing, place the yoghurt, ginger, turmeric and salt in a small bowl and mix to combine.

To serve, divide rice, edamame, cucumber and radish between 4 bowls. Top with sliced chicken, dressing and coriander sprigs.
SERVES 4

Talk about TICKING BOXES – *this bowl is full of absolute goodness* and tastes as amazing as it looks. No wonder it's my NEW FAVE *go-to dinner.*

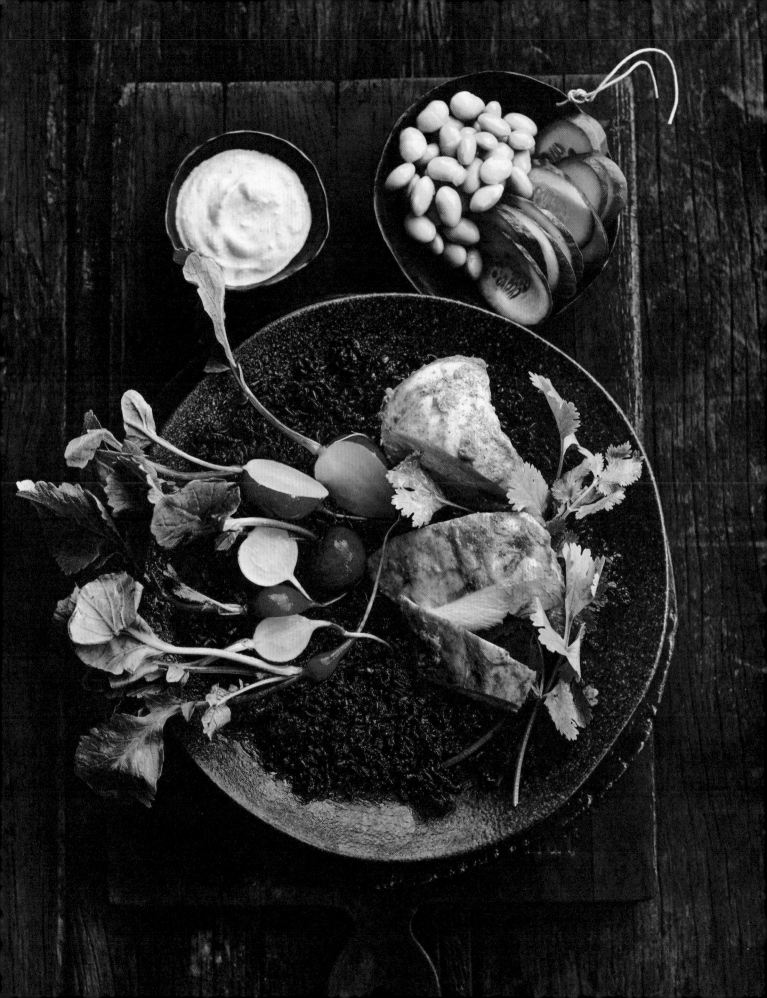

tom's PUMPKIN
salad *bowl*

1 small Japanese pumpkin
2 tablespoons extra virgin olive oil
2 tablespoons pure maple syrup
sea salt and cracked black pepper
100g (3½ oz) baby spinach leaves
100g (3½ oz) baby rocket (arugula) leaves
1 small red onion, thinly sliced
2 tablespoons pomegranate molasses or balsamic glaze
200g (7oz) marinated feta
½ cup (80g/2¾ oz) chopped roasted almonds
8 slices prosciutto (optional)

Preheat oven to 200°C (400°C).
  Cut the pumpkin in half horizontally. Scoop out and discard seeds so you have 2 large bowls.
  Place the pumpkin, cut-side up, on a baking tray lined with non-stick baking paper. Drizzle with oil and maple and sprinkle with salt and pepper. Bake for 50 minutes or until the pumpkin is soft.
  In a large bowl, combine the spinach, rocket, onion and molasses.
  To serve, place the pumpkin on a serving platter. Add the salad to the pumpkin bowls. Serve topped with crumbled feta, almonds and prosciutto, if you like. **SERVES 4**

MY SON made this for me after watching something similar on his computer. *It was seriously delicious!* He was SO PROUD of his efforts.
I had a total proud mother moment too!

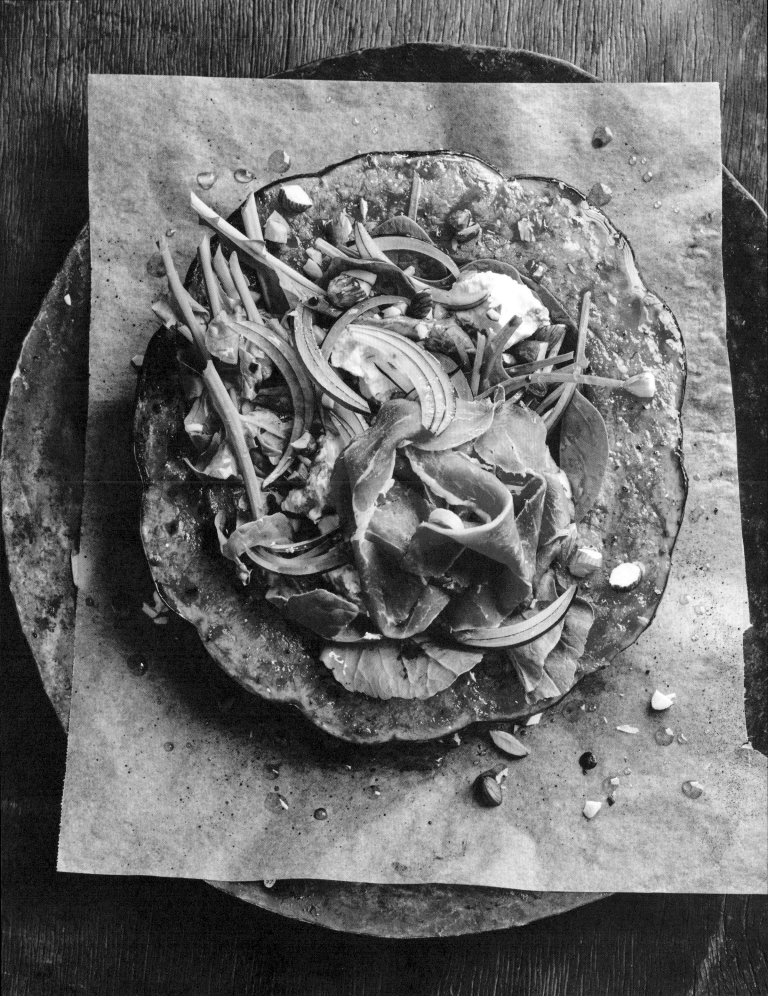

kale AND pumpkin falafels
with pickled carrot slaw

¾ cup (120g/4½ oz) toasted pepitas (pumpkin seeds)
3 cups (90g/3 oz) shredded kale, stems removed
   (about 3 large leaves)
1 clove garlic, crushed
1 x 400g (1 lb) can chickpeas (garbanzo beans), rinsed, drained
1½ teaspoons ground turmeric
½ cup (6g/¼ oz) coriander (cilantro) leaves
sea salt and cracked black pepper
3 cups (450g/1 lb) firmly packed grated pumpkin
extra virgin olive oil, for brushing
plain Greek-style (thick) yoghurt and hulled tahini, to serve
pickled carrot slaw
6 carrots, shredded using a julienne peeler
2 tablespoons apple cider vinegar
2 tablespoons honey
2 large red chillies, sliced
½ cup (6g/¼ oz) coriander (cilantro) leaves

Preheat oven to 220°C (425°F).
   Place the pepitas into the bowl of a food processor and process until finely chopped. Add the kale, garlic, chickpeas, turmeric, coriander, salt and pepper and process until well combined. Add the pumpkin and stir through to combine.
   Shape large tablespoonfuls of pumpkin mixture into balls. Place on a baking tray lined with non-stick baking paper and flatten slightly. Brush well with oil, then bake for 25 minutes or until golden and crisp.
   To make the pickled carrot slaw, place the carrots, vinegar, honey, chilli and coriander in a bowl and toss to combine. Set aside for 5 minutes to pickle.
   To serve, divide the pickled carrot slaw between bowls and top with pumpkin falafels and serve with yoghurt and tahini. **SERVES 4**

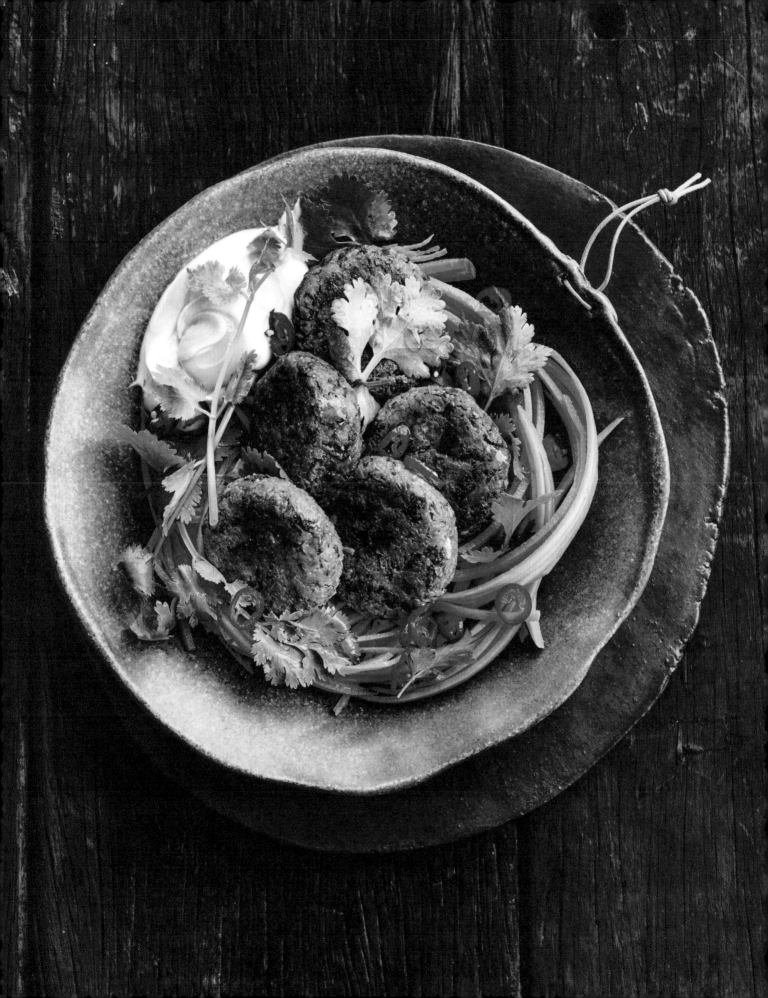

poached LIME CHICKEN
and fennel slaw *with*
coconut dressing

2 x 200g (7 oz) chicken breast fillets, trimmed

4 cups (1 litre/34 fl oz) chicken stock

2 cups (500ml/17 fl oz) water

2 lemongrass stalks, halved and bruised

1 green chilli, halved

4 kaffir lime leaves, bruised

4cm (1½ inch) piece ginger, sliced

purple shiso leaves, to serve (optional)

coconut dressing

1 cup (250ml/8½ fl oz) coconut cream

2 tablespoons lime juice

2 tablespoons fish sauce

1 tablespoon caster (superfine) sugar

fennel slaw

3 medium fennel bulbs, thinly sliced

2 Lebanese cucumbers, thinly sliced

2 cups (24g/1 oz) coriander (cilantro) leaves

⅓ cup (5g/¼ oz) mint leaves

1 green chilli, thinly sliced

Halve chicken breasts through the centre to make 2 even pieces.

Place stock, water, lemongrass, chilli, kaffir lime and ginger in a medium saucepan and bring to the boil. Reduce heat and simmer for 10 minutes. Add chicken and return to boil for 1 minute. Cover with a tight-fitting lid. Turn off heat and poach in liquid for 10 minutes. Allow to cool slightly and use 2 forks to shred into large pieces.

To make the coconut dressing, place the coconut cream, lime juice, fish sauce and sugar in a bowl and stir to combine.

To make the fennel slaw, place the fennel, cucumber, coriander, mint and chilli in a large bowl. Add shredded chicken and dressing and toss lightly to combine. Divide between bowls and sprinkle with shiso leaves to serve. **SERVES 4**

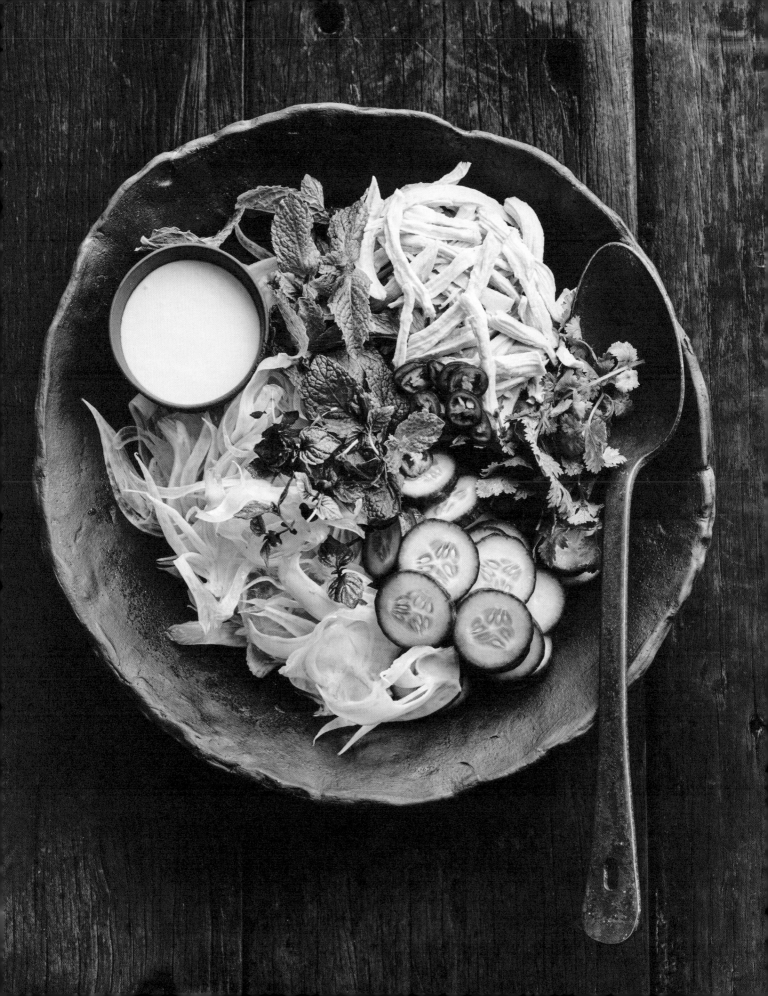

asian BEEF SKEWERS
with *coconut noodle bowls*

500g (1 lb 1 oz) grass-fed beef fillet, trimmed and cut into strips
2 tablespoons fish sauce
2 tablespoons lime juice
1 tablespoon brown sugar
2 cloves garlic, crushed
1 tablespoon finely grated ginger
2 green onions (scallions), finely chopped
extra virgin olive oil, for brushing
400g (14 oz) snow peas (mange tout), blanched and
   sliced lengthways
coriander (cilantro), roasted peanuts and sliced green chilli,
   to serve
coconut noodles
200g (7 oz) dried rice noodles
½ cup (125ml/4¼ fl oz) coconut cream
2 tablespoons lime juice
2 tablespoons fish sauce
1 tablespoon caster (superfine) sugar

Place the beef, fish sauce, lime juice, brown sugar, garlic, ginger and onion into a bowl and toss to combine. Set aside for 10 minutes then thread onto skewers.

Heat a char-grill pan or barbecue over high heat.

Brush the beef skewers with oil and char-grill for 3 minutes each side or until golden and charred. Set aside.

To make the coconut noodles, pour boiling water over the noodles and stand for 4 minutes or until softened, then drain and rinse under cold running water. Place the coconut cream, lime juice, fish sauce and sugar into a bowl stir to combine. Add the drained rice noodles to the coconut sauce.

Place the noodles with sauce into a bowl and top with the snow peas, coriander, peanuts and chilli. Serve topped with the beef skewers. **SERVES 4**

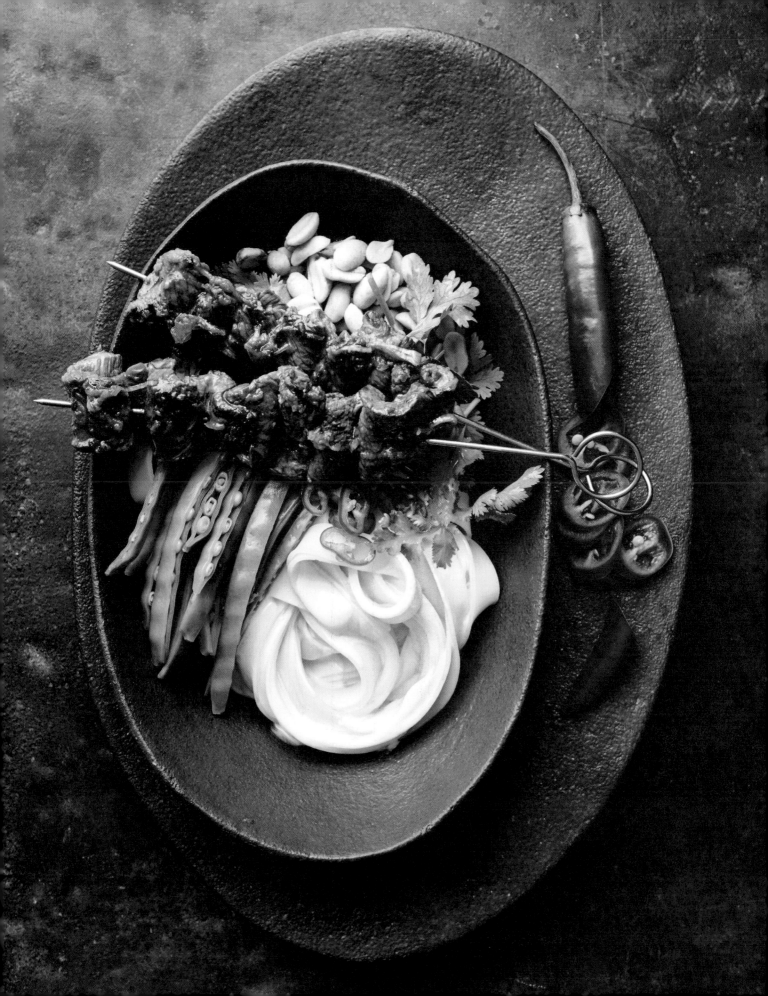

celery SALAD with *bloody mary dressing*

4 oxheart or heirloom tomatoes

6 radishes, thinly sliced using a mandoline

4 small celery stalks, peeled into ribbons

2 cups (48g/1½ oz) baby celery leaves

180g (6½ oz) haloumi, shaved

16 green olives

2 medium dill pickles, sliced

Bloody Mary dressing

½ cup (125ml/4¼ oz) tomato puree (passata)

2 teaspoons Worcestershire sauce

2 teaspoons lemon juice

1 tablespoon vodka (optional)

1 teaspoon Tabasco sauce

sea salt and cracked black pepper

To make the Bloody Mary dressing, place the tomato puree, Worcestershire sauce, lemon juice, vodka, Tabasco, salt and pepper in a small bowl. Mix to combine and set aside.

Slice the tomatoes across the width into 1.5 cm (½ inch) thick rounds. To serve, place the tomatoes on a platter and top with radishes, celery ribbons, celery leaves, haloumi, olives and pickles. Drizzle with the Bloody Mary dressing. **SERVES 4**

This UPSIDE-DOWN version of a Bloody Mary makes the perfect salad – loads of CRUNCH with just *the right amount of dressing kick!*

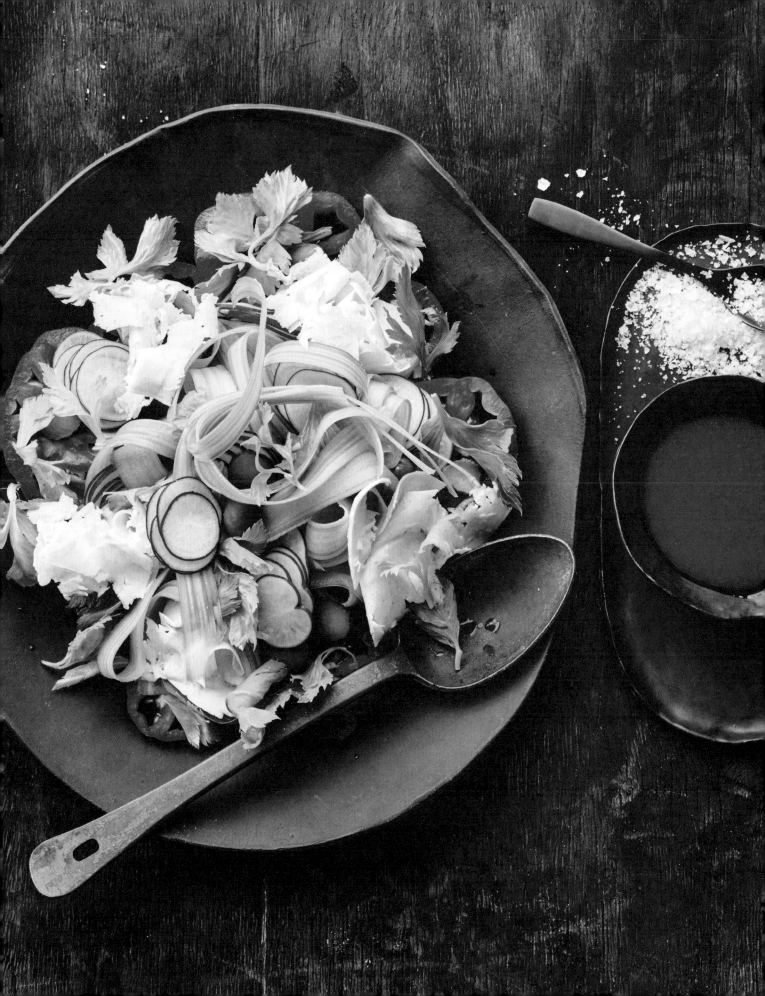

coconut AND ginger rice bowls with *salmon*

4 cups (800g/1 lb 12 oz) cooked brown rice, at room temperature
450g (1 lb) skinless sashimi-grade salmon fillet, cut into cubes
3 celery stalks, shaved with a peeler
1 avocado, peeled, seed removed and quartered
1 cup (140g/4¼ oz) frozen shelled edamame beans, blanched
shredded nori sheets and pickled ginger, to serve
coconut dressing
¾ cup (180ml/6 fl oz) coconut cream
¼ cup (70g/2½ oz) pickled ginger, finely chopped
2 teaspoons finely grated lime rind
2 tablespoons lime juice
1 large green chilli, thinly sliced

To make the coconut dressing, combine the coconut cream, pickled ginger, lime rind and juice and chilli in a small bowl.

To serve, stir ½ the coconut dressing through the rice and divide between serving bowls. Top with the salmon, celery, avocado, edamame beans, nori and pickled ginger. Serve with the remaining coconut dressing. **SERVES 4**

You can *swap the salmon for tuna*, kingfish or ocean trout. For a VEGETARIAN option, *silken firm tofu teams well* with the Asian flavours.

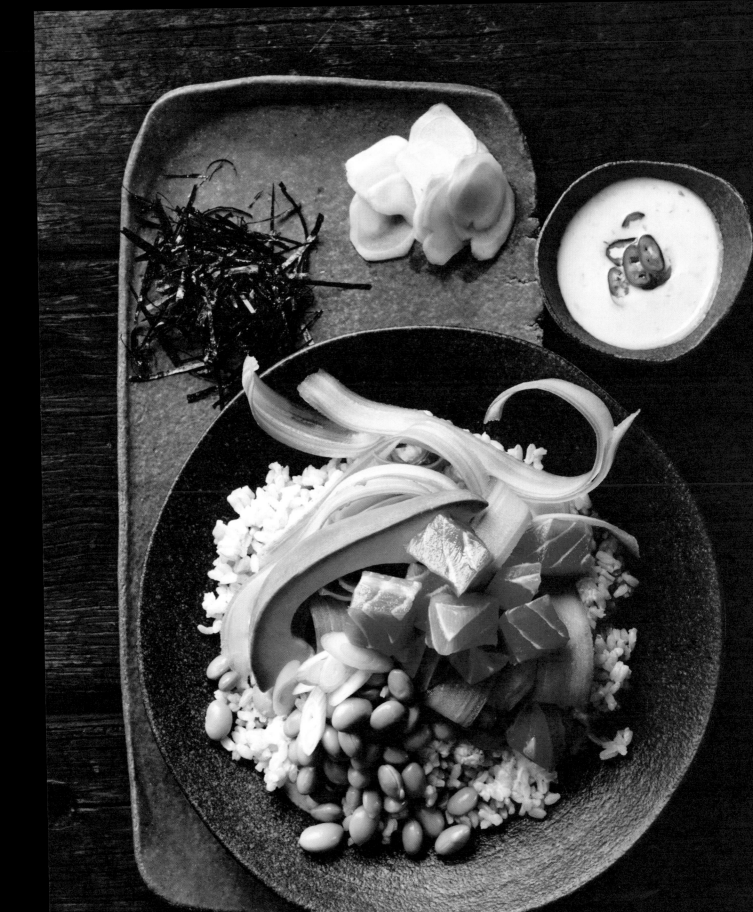

miso ROASTED brussels sprouts *salad bowl*

700g (1 lb 5 oz) medium Brussels sprouts, trimmed, halved
4 cups (800g/1 lb 8 oz) cooked black rice
2 bulbs baby fennel, shaved using a mandoline, to serve
1 cup (25g/¾ oz) red-veined sorrel leaves, to serve
maple miso marinade
2 tablespoons white miso paste (shiro)
2 tablespoons pure maple syrup
1 tablespoon mirin (Japanese rice wine)
2 teaspoons sesame oil
2 tablespoons black sesame seeds
pickled radish
½ cup (125ml/4¼ oz) rice wine vinegar
2 teaspoons caster (superfine) sugar
pinch sea salt flakes
6 radishes, thinly sliced using a mandolin

Preheat oven to 220°C (425°F).
    Place the Brussels sprouts in a large bowl and set aside.
    To make the maple miso marinade, in a small bowl, whisk together miso, maple, mirin and oil until a smooth consistency. Mix through sesame seeds. Pour marinade over sprouts and toss to combine.
    Spread marinated sprouts in an even layer on a baking tray lined with non-stick baking paper. Roast for 20 minutes or until golden and caramelised.
    To make the pickled radish, combine vinegar, sugar and salt in a medium bowl and whisk until sugar and salt has dissolved. Add sliced radish to the bowl and set aside for 10 minutes.
    To serve, divide rice between serving bowls. Top with roasted sprouts, fennel and pickled radish. Garnish with sorrel and drizzle with remaining pickling liquid. **SERVES 4**

If you don't like Brussels sprouts then *this recipe will change your mind* – roasted in miso and maple, these CRUNCHY DELIGHTS take on a whole new persona and are *hard to resist.*

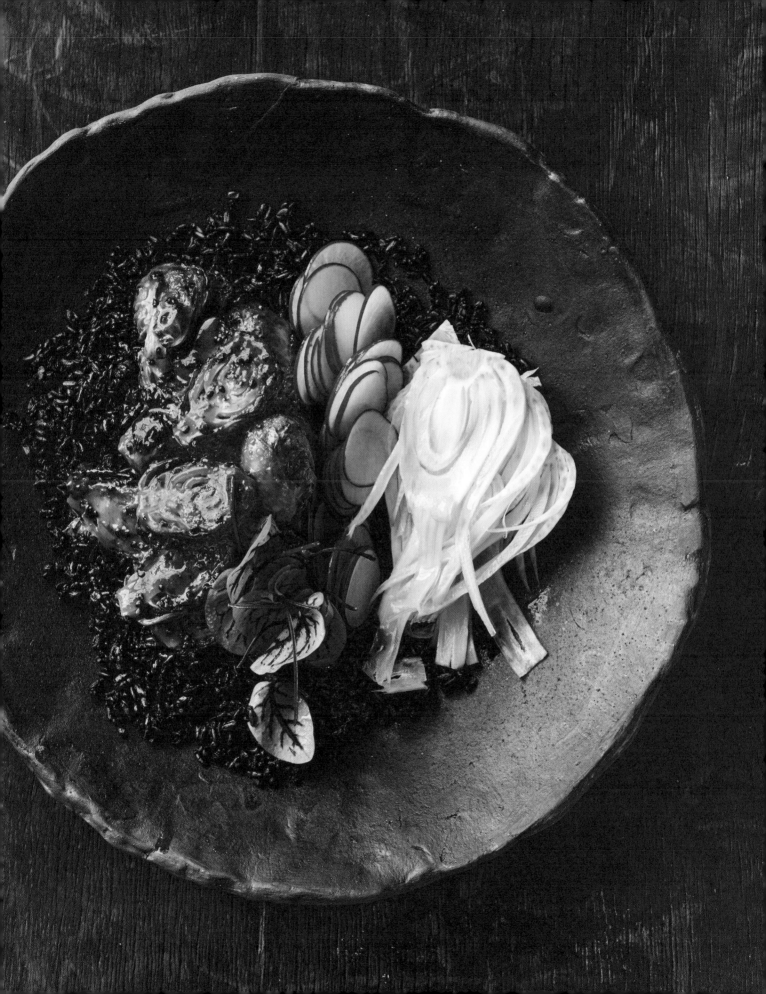

eggplant
BABA GHANOUSH *bowl*

4 x 350g (12¼ oz) medium eggplants (aubergines)
2 tablespoons extra virgin olive oil
sea salt and cracked black pepper
baba ghanoush
1 clove garlic
2 tablespoons hulled tahini
1 cup (280g/10 oz) plain Greek-style (thick) yoghurt
juice of ½ lemon
¼ cup (60ml/2 fl oz) extra virgin olive oil
sea salt and cracked black pepper
freekeh salad
2 cups (320g/11¼ oz) cooked freekeh
1 green onion (scallion), finely sliced
2 cucumbers, sliced into rounds
1 cup (24g/¾ oz) flat-leaf parsley leaves
1 cup (16g/½ oz) mint leaves
extra virgin olive oil, sea salt and cracked black pepper, to taste

Preheat oven to 200°C (400°F).

Slice eggplants in half down the length and score flesh into a diamond pattern, being careful not to go through the skin. Brush with oil and season with salt and pepper. Place, cut-side up, on a baking tray lined with non-stick baking paper. Bake for 40 minutes or until flesh is soft and caramelised.

To make the baba ghanoush, scoop half the flesh from the middle of each eggplant 'bowl' and set aside to cool for 10 minutes. Once cool, blitz in a food processor along with the garlic, tahini, yoghurt and lemon juice. With the motor running, slowly drizzle in oil and season with salt and pepper.

To make the freekeh salad, place the freekeh, green onion, cucumber, parsley and mint in a bowl and toss to combine. Drizzle with oil and season with salt and pepper.

To serve, place 2 eggplant 'bowls' onto each serving plate. Fill with baba ghanoush and top with freekeh salad. **SERVES 4**

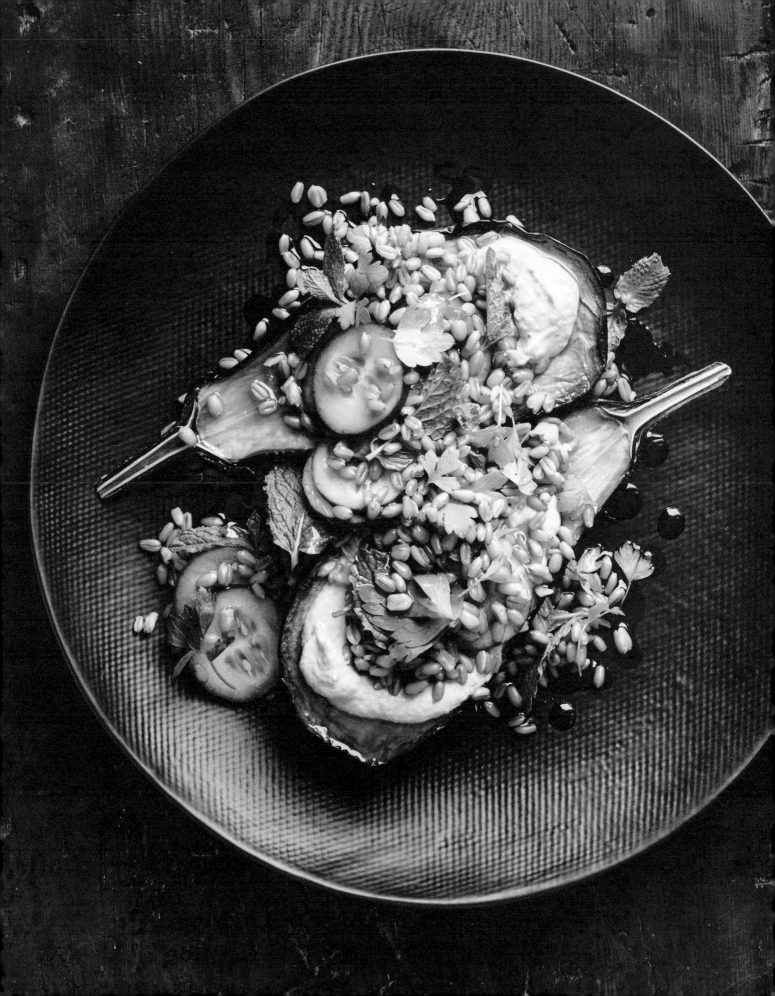

spaghetti SQUASH BOWLS with *haloumi croutons*

2 x 1.4kg (3 lb 1 oz) spaghetti squash
2 tablespoons extra virgin olive oil
sea salt and cracked black pepper
haloumi croutons
1 tablespoon extra virgin olive oil
300g (10½ oz) haloumi, cut into 3cm (1¼ inch) cubes
1 cup (100g/3½ oz) walnuts, roughly chopped
2 cups (60g/2 oz) shredded cavolo nero (Tuscan kale)
½ cup (8g/½ oz) sage leaves
⅓ cup (80ml/2¾ fl oz) lemon juice
2 tablespoons honey
sea salt and cracked black pepper

Preheat oven to 200°C (400°F).

Cut spaghetti squash in half lengthwise then, using a spoon, scrape away and discard seeds. Place squash, cut-side down, on a baking tray lined with non-stick baking paper. Roast for 45 minutes or until the flesh is soft.

While the spaghetti squash is cooking, make the haloumi croutons. Heat a medium frying pan over medium-high heat. Add the oil and haloumi and cook for 5 minutes or until golden on all sides. Add the walnuts, cavolo nero and sage. Cook for a further 5 minutes or until walnuts are toasted and cavolo nero is wilted. Remove from heat and add the lemon juice, honey, salt and pepper.

Once the squash is cooked, drizzle flesh with oil and season with salt and pepper. Use a fork to scrape the flesh into 'spaghetti' strands.

To serve, divide filling between each squash half and gently toss to combine. **SERVES 4**

SALTY, SWEET and delicious! *These golden spaghetti squash* are like MAGIC the way they transform themselves.

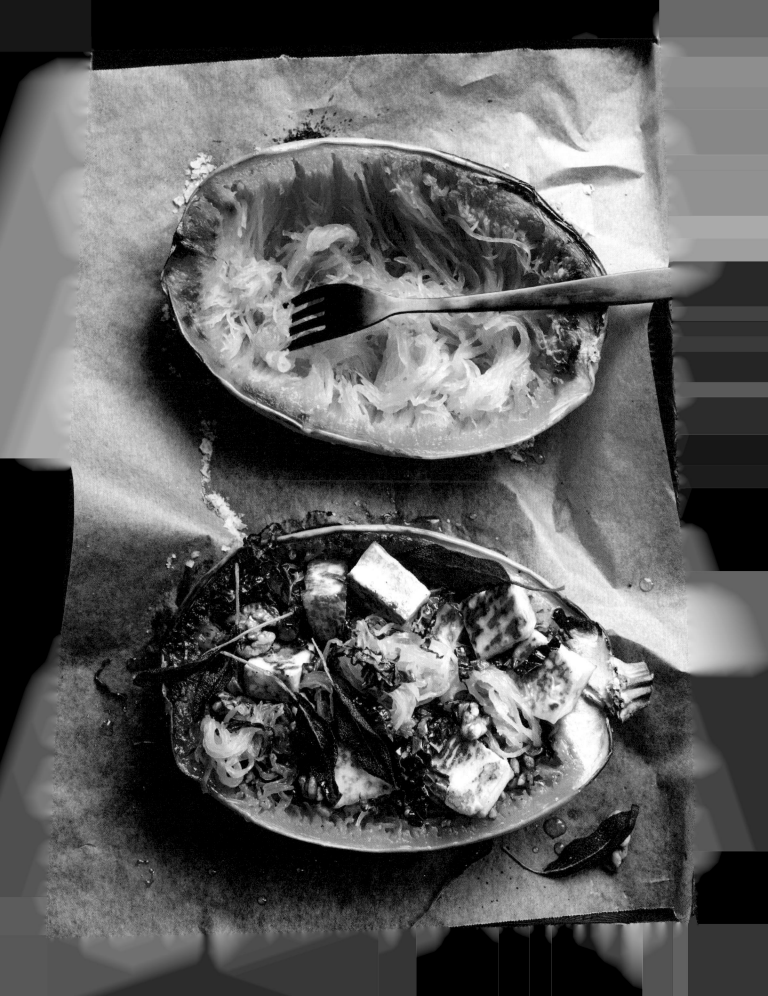

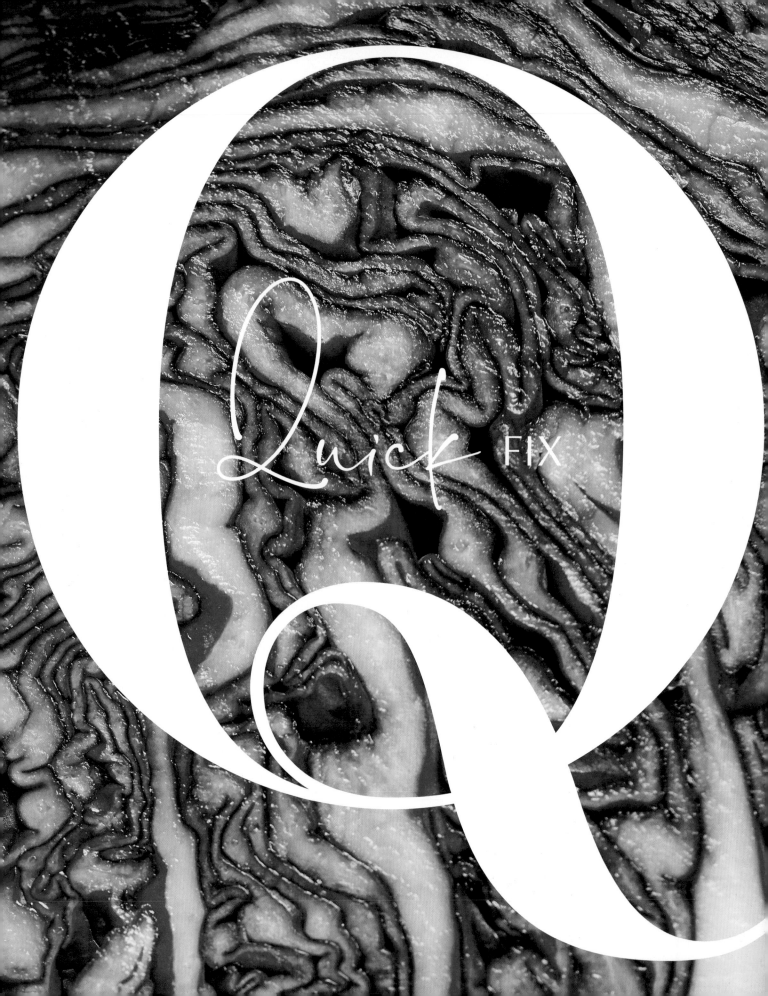

Quick FIX

Sometimes, life gets hectic. There's no use pretending, *for me it's most days!* That's why I'm always on the hunt for SMARTER, FASTER ways to make simply delicious meals using everyday ingredients and MAKING THEM SHINE. These will be your saviours, when you're under the pump or on the run. *Introducing, your new weeknight favourites.*

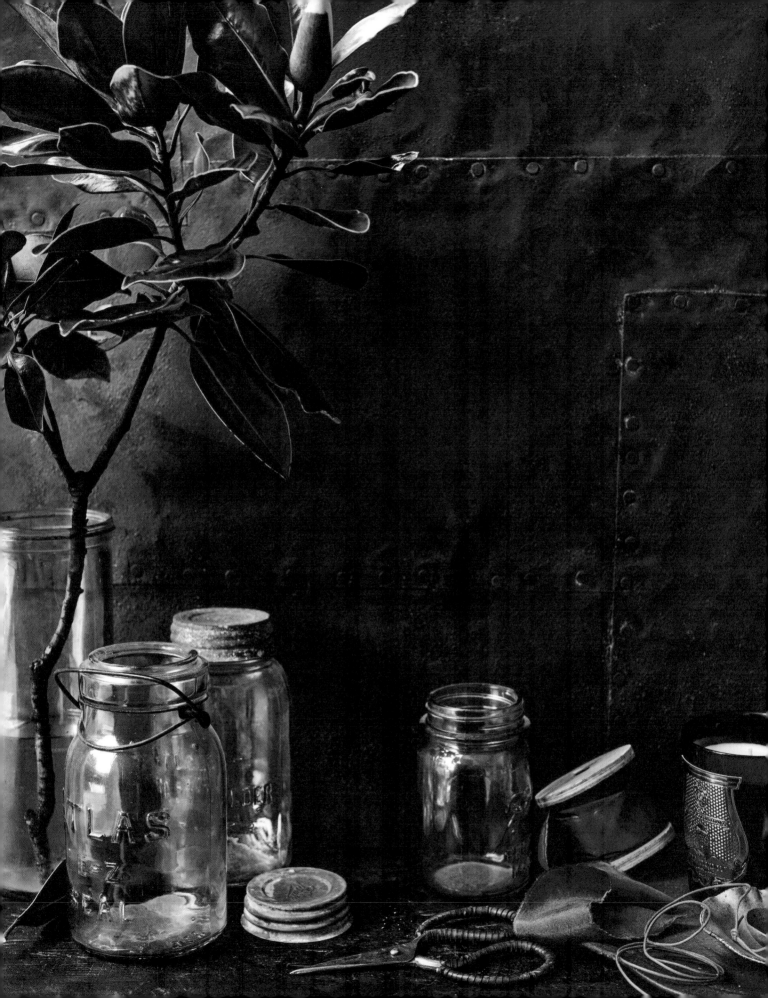

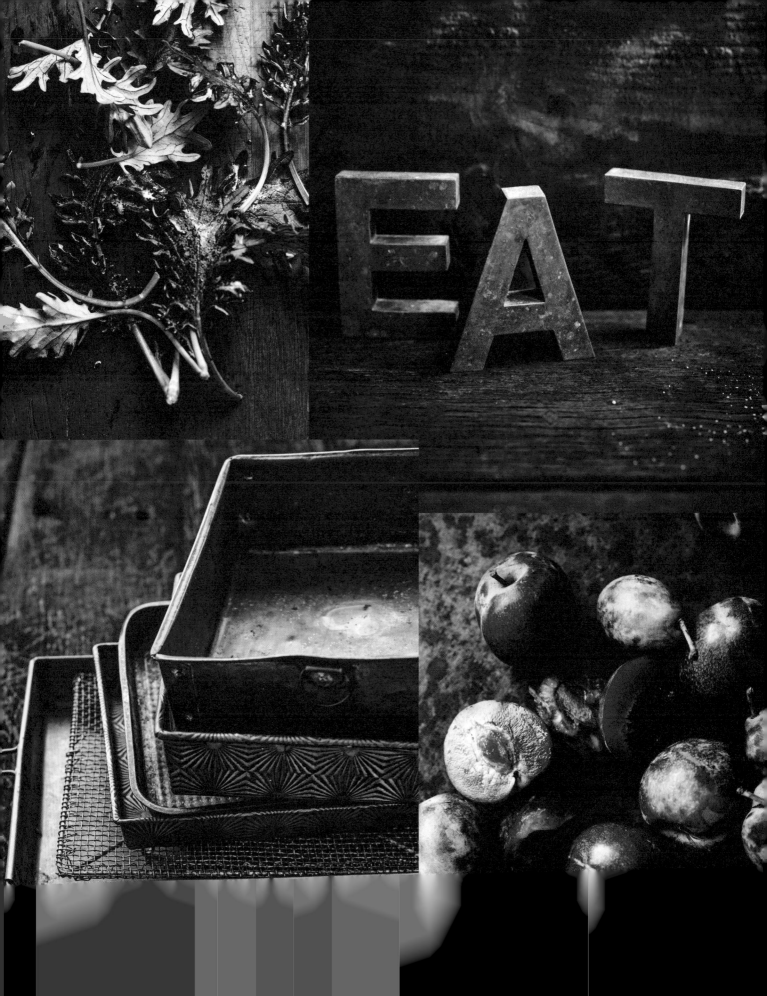

chorizo AND cauliflower *bolognese*

2 fresh chorizo sausages (casings removed), finely chopped
2 cloves garlic, crushed
2 tablespoons oregano leaves
1 tablespoon extra virgin olive oil
600g (1 lb 3 oz) cauliflower, finely chopped
cracked black pepper
1 x 400g (14 oz) can crushed tomatoes
½ cup (125ml/4¼ fl oz) beef stock
3 zucchini (courgettes), shredded using a julienne peeler
200g (7 oz) dried wholemeal (whole-wheat) spaghetti, cooked
finely grated parmesan and fresh mozzarella, to serve

Heat a large frying pan over medium-high heat. Add the chorizo, garlic
and oregano. Cook, stirring occasionally, for 5 minutes or until golden.
Remove from pan.
   Add oil, cauliflower and pepper to the frying pan and cook for
8 minutes or until cauliflower has softened and is just starting
to brown. Return the chorizo mixture back to the pan and stir to
combine. Add the tomato and stock. Reduce heat and simmer rapidly
for 5 minutes.
   Spoon the bolognese over the zucchini noodles and warm pasta.
Serve with a sprinkling of parmesan and a piece of fresh mozzarella.
SERVES 4

Classic bolognese lovers will be easily converted
to this UPFLAVOURED version – *the kick of
chorizo* with all the deliciousness of golden
cauliflower in a RICH TOMATO sauce. *Yes please!*

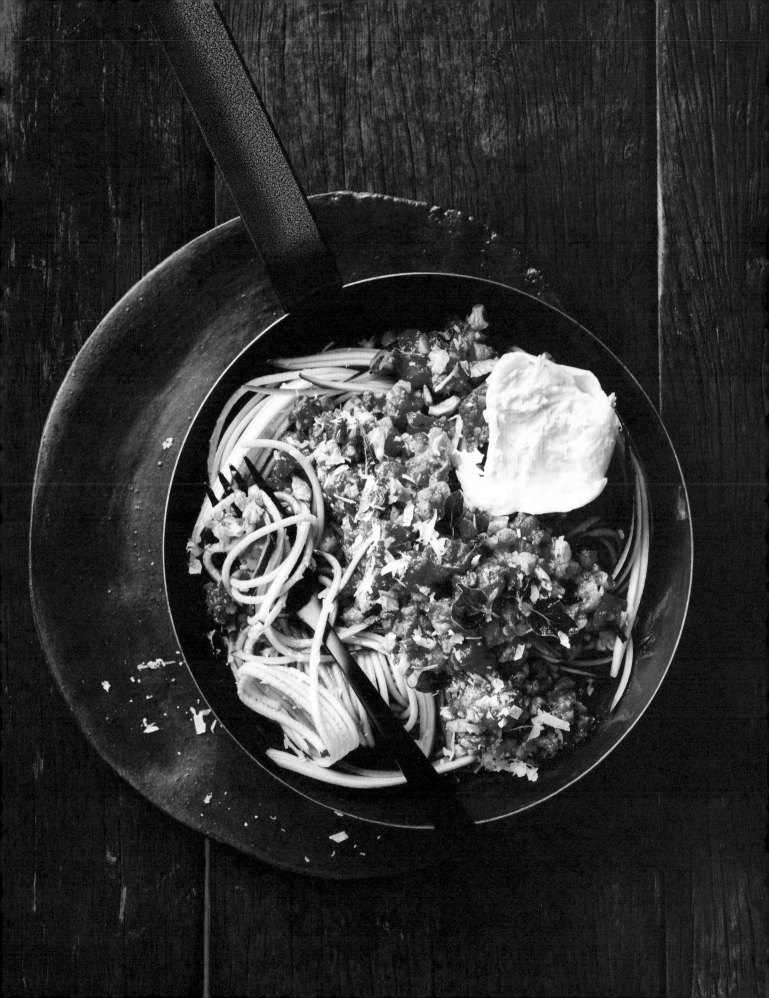

tarragon ROASTED MUSHROOMS with *cashew sauce*

⅓ cup (80ml/2¾ fl oz) extra virgin olive oil
¼ cup (8g/¼ oz) tarragon leaves, roughly chopped
16 portobello or large Swiss brown mushrooms, halved
2 red onions, sliced into wedges
grilled flatbreads and baby kale, to serve
cashew sauce
1 cup (150g/5¼ oz) raw cashews
½ cup (125ml/4¼ fl oz) water
1 tablespoon tamari
2 tablespoons lemon juice
1 tablespoon nutritional yeast

Preheat oven to 220°C (425°F).

To make the cashew sauce, place the cashews in a bowl and cover with boiling water. Allow to stand for 20 minutes and drain. Place the cashews, water, tamari, lemon juice and nutritional yeast in a blender and blend until smooth. Allow to stand for 10 minutes for the flavours to come together.

In a small bowl, place the oil and tarragon and mix to combine. Set aside.

Thread 4 mushroom halves and red onion wedges onto skewers, alternating between each. Place skewers on a baking tray lined with non-stick baking paper and brush with the tarragon oil. Bake skewers for 10 minutes. Brush again with the tarragon oil and bake for a further 10 minutes or until the mushrooms are a deep golden colour.

To serve, divide the grilled flatbreads between plates and top with cashew sauce and roasted mushroom skewers. Serve with baby kale.

MAKES 8 SKEWERS

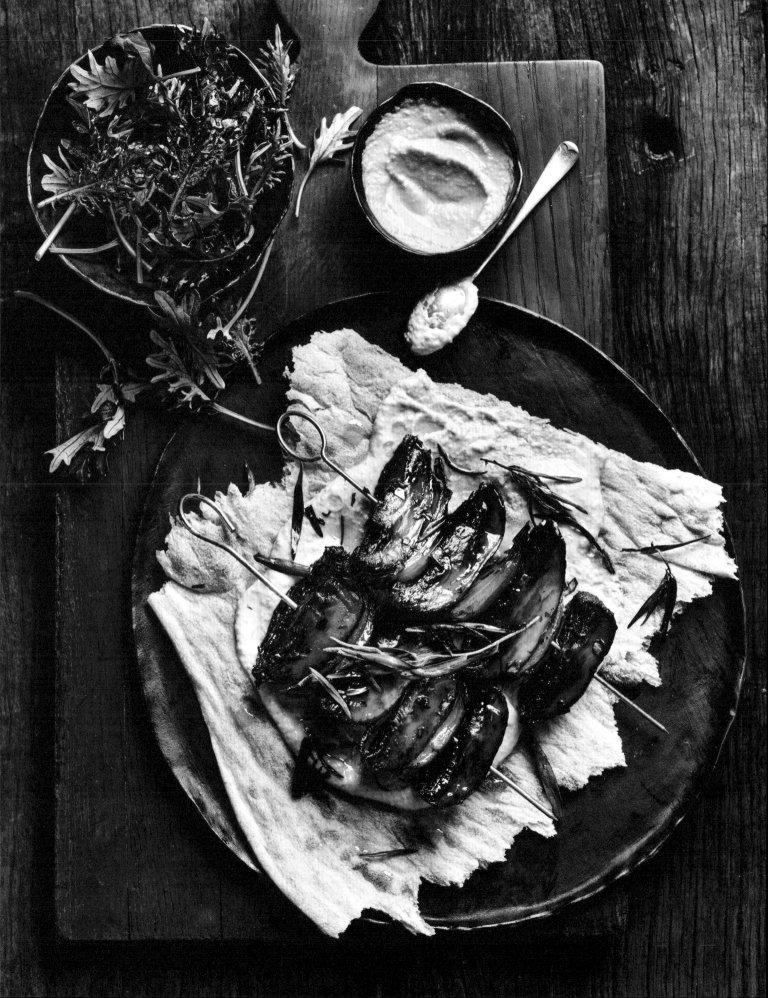

harissa GRILLED SALMON
with *leeks*

3 leeks, halved lengthways
2 tablespoons extra virgin olive oil
sea salt and cracked black pepper
1 tablespoon harissa paste
1 tablespoon honey
450g (1 lb) piece skinless salmon fillet, pin boned
green salad and lime cheeks, to serve

Preheat oven to 220°C (425°F).
   Place the leeks, cut-side up, on a baking tray lined with non-stick
baking paper. Drizzle with oil and sprinkle with salt and pepper.
Bake for 20–25 minutes or until soft and lightly golden.
   Increase oven temperature to 240°C (465°F).
   Combine the harissa and honey and spread over the top of the
salmon. Place the salmon on top of the leeks and bake for 10 minutes
or until the salmon is golden and cooked to your liking.
   Serve the salmon with the leeks, a simple green salad and a squeeze
of lime. **SERVES 4**

With a VIBRANT hit of harissa, *this recipe works
with any firm fish fillet*. Feel free to choose
whatever's SUSTAINABLE and local to you.

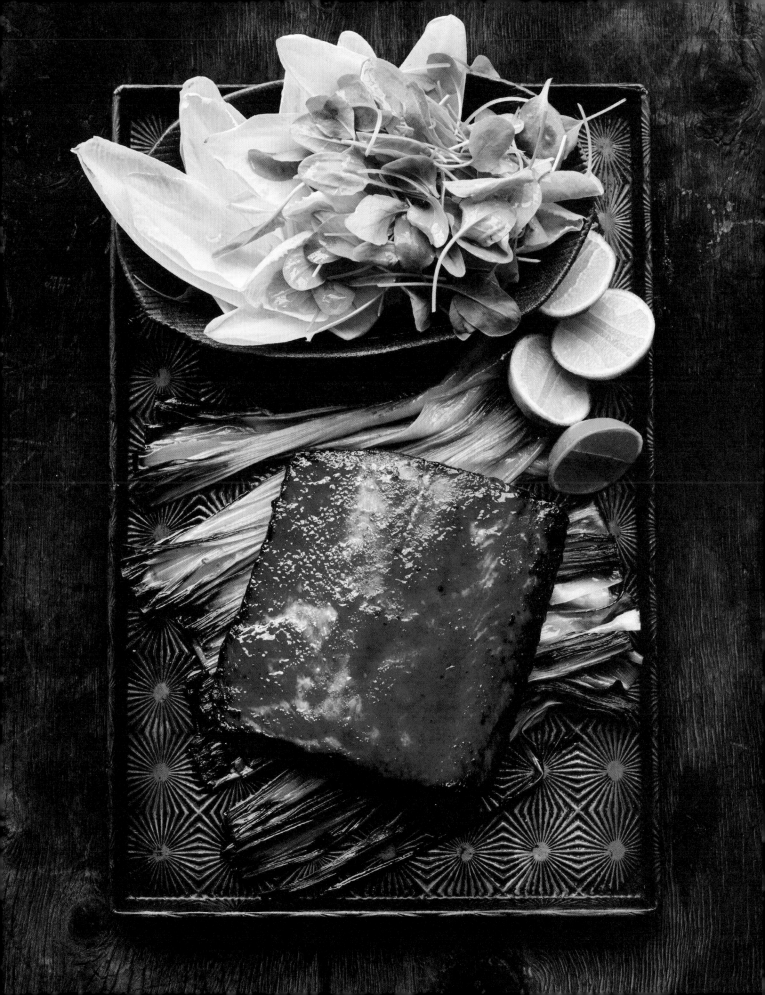

cauliflower AND TAHINI PATTIES with *whipped goat's cheese*

3 cucumbers, thinly sliced into ribbons
baby mint, ground sumac and lemon cheeks, to serve
cauliflower and tahini patties
1 x 400g (14 oz) can chickpeas (garbanzo beans), drained and peeled
500g (1 lb 1 oz) cauliflower
1 clove garlic, crushed
1½ teaspoons ground cumin
½ cup (12g/½ oz) chopped flat-leaf parsley leaves
¼ cup (60ml/2 fl oz) apple cider vinegar
3 green onions (scallions), finely sliced
1 cup (280g/10 oz) hulled tahini
sea salt and cracked black pepper
extra virgin olive oil, for brushing and drizzling
whipped goat's cheese
160g (5½ oz) soft goat's cheese
1 cup (280g/10 oz) plain Greek-style (thick) yoghurt

Preheat oven to 220°C (425°F).

To make the cauliflower and tahini patties, place the chickpeas in a bowl and mash well. Grate the cauliflower on a box grater so it is finely chopped (you should have 3 cups of firmly packed cauliflower). Add the cauliflower, garlic, cumin, parsley, vinegar, onion, tahini, salt and pepper to the chickpeas and mix well to combine. Shape ¼ cupfuls into small patties and place on a baking tray lined with non-stick baking paper. Brush with oil and bake for 15 minutes then brush again with extra oil and bake for a further 10 minutes or until golden.

To make the whipped goat's cheese, place the goat's cheese and 1 tablespoon of the yoghurt in a small bowl and mix to combine. Add remaining yoghurt and whisk until smooth.

To serve, divide cauliflower and tahini patties and the whipped goat's cheese between plates. Drizzle the whipped goat's cheese with oil and top with cucumber and baby mint. Sprinkle with sumac and serve with a squeeze of lemon. **SERVES 4**

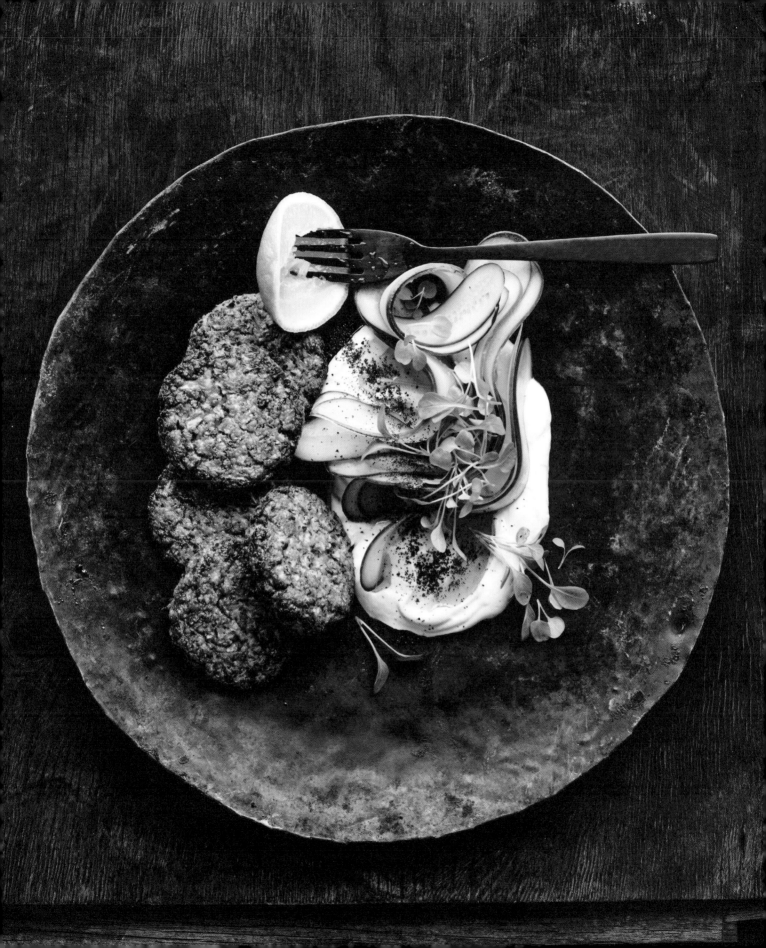

Tuna AND soba *noodle bowl*

375g (13 oz) sashimi-grade tuna
2 teaspoons wasabi paste
1–2 nori sheets
vegetable oil, for brushing
180g (4 oz) dried soba noodles, cooked, drained and kept warm
12 baby purple carrots, cleaned, blanched and halved
pickled ginger and baby purple shiso leaves, to serve
soy dressing
¼ cup (60ml/2 fl oz) lime juice
2 tablespoons soy sauce
1½ tablespoons mirin (Japanese rice wine)

Sparingly spread all sides of the tuna with the wasabi paste and wrap in a sheet of nori to enclose, trimming any excess nori.

Heat a non-stick frying pan over medium-high heat. Lightly brush the nori with oil and cook the tuna for 20–30 seconds each side or until seared. Set aside for 5 minutes before slicing.

To make the soy dressing, place the lime juice, soy and mirin in a bowl and mix to combine.

To serve, divide the noodles, carrot and tuna between serving bowls. Spoon over the dressing and serve with pickled ginger and shiso leaves. **SERVES 4**

If you can't get your hands on *a piece of tuna,* try kingfish or salmon. Apart from fish, *beef eye fillet will also team well* with the PUNCHY *Japanese flavours.*

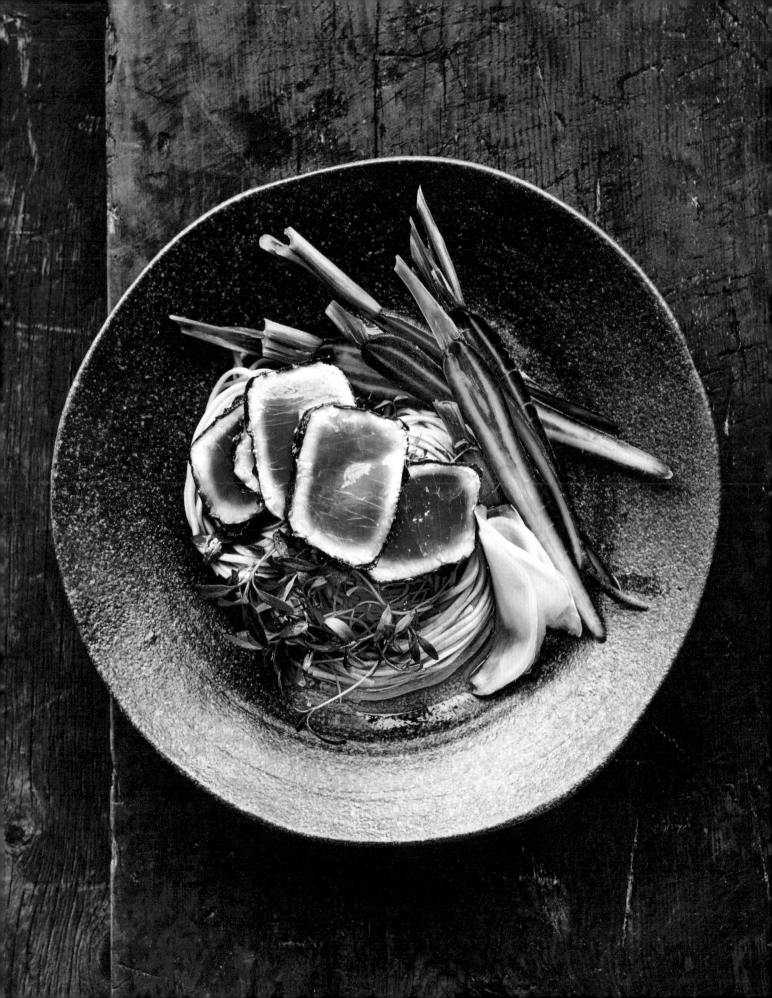

spiced CHICKPEA BALLS with *herbed zucchini salad*

spiced chickpea balls

3 carrots, peeled and chopped

1 x 400g (14 oz) can chickpeas (garbanzo beans), drained

½ cup (120g/4¼ oz) fresh ricotta

½ cup (6g/¼ oz) coriander (cilantro) leaves

1 teaspoon ground cumin

2 teaspoons finely grated ginger

1 clove garlic, crushed

2 tablespoons white chia seeds

sesame seeds, for rolling

extra virgin olive oil, for brushing

herbed zucchini salad

3 zucchini (courgettes), shredded using a julienne peeler

1 pomegranate, seeds removed

1 cup (24g/¾ oz) flat-leaf parsley leaves

½ cup (8g/¼ oz) mint leaves

2 tablespoons extra virgin olive oil

1 tablespoon lemon juice

sea salt and cracked black pepper

Preheat oven 180°C (350°F).

To make the spiced chickpea balls, place carrot in the bowl of a food processor and process until finely chopped. Add the chickpeas, ricotta, coriander, cumin, ginger, garlic and chia seeds and process until combined. Roll small tablespoonfuls of mixture into balls, roll in sesame seeds and place on a baking tray lined with non-stick baking paper. Brush with oil and bake for 20 minutes or until golden.

While the chickpea balls are cooking, make the herbed zucchini salad. In a bowl, add zucchini, pomegranate seeds, parsley, mint, oil and lemon juice and toss to combine. Season with salt and pepper to taste.

To serve, divide the salad and balls between plates. **SERVES 4**

The beauty of this dish is that it makes for the most amazing PORTABLE PICNIC or lunch. *Simply pile the salad* and balls onto pita or FLATBREADS and *away you go!*

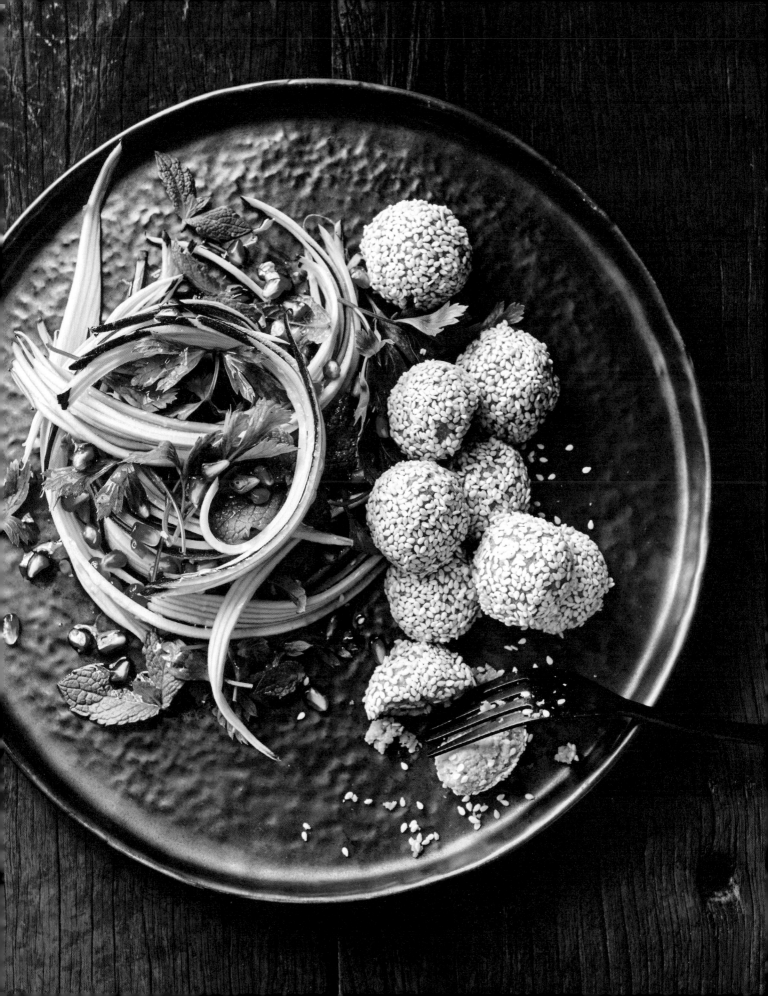

grilled EGGPLANTS WITH *roasted garlic yoghurt and broad beans*

3 x 330g (11½ oz) small eggplants (aubergines), cut into wedges
140g (1½ oz) rocket (arugula) (about 1 bunch), trimmed
2 cups (300g/10½ oz) frozen broad beans, blanched and peeled
extra virgin olive oil and lemon cheeks, to serve
roasted garlic yoghurt
1 bulb garlic
1 cup (280g/10 oz) plain Greek-style (thick) yoghurt
sea salt and cracked black pepper

Preheat oven to 180°C (350°F).

To make the roasted garlic yoghurt, wrap the garlic in aluminium foil and place on a baking tray. Bake for 45 minutes or until soft. Set aside to cool slightly. Squeeze the garlic from the skins and place into a bowl. Mash the garlic until smooth. Add the yoghurt, salt and pepper and mix to combine.

To grill the eggplants, heat a char-grill pan or barbecue grill over medium-high heat. Char-grill the eggplant for 5 minutes on all 3 sides or until soft.

To serve, place the roasted garlic yoghurt onto serving plates and top with the eggplant, rocket and broad beans. Drizzle with oil and serve with lemon cheeks. **SERVES 4**

This is my version of BABA GHANOUSH *if it wanted to be a chunky salad* – all the wonderful flavours with more bite and FRESHNESS.

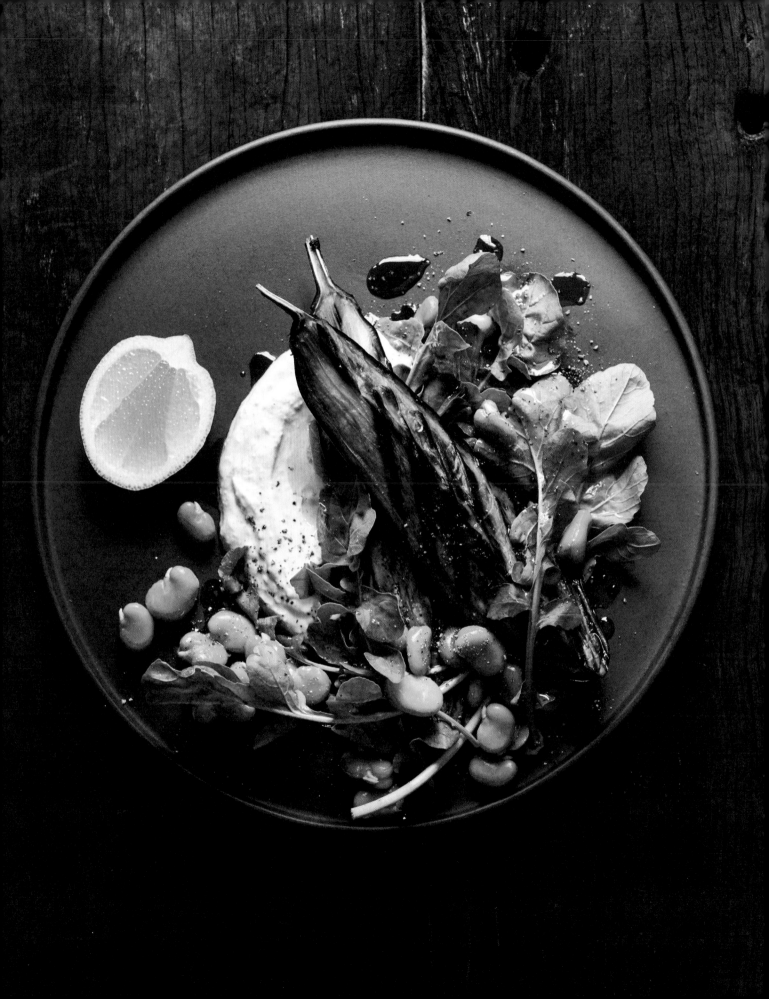

sesame AND NORI CRISP FISH
with *japanese slaw*

4 sheets nori, finely shredded with scissors
¼ cup (40g/1½ oz) sesame seeds
1 teaspoon sea salt flakes, crushed
4 x 150g (5¼ oz) skinless firm white fish fillets[+]
1 tablespoon grapeseed oil or vegetable oil
1 tablespoon toasted sesame seeds, to serve
sesame dressing
¼ cup (70g/2½ oz) hulled tahini
2 tablespoons rice wine vinegar
2 tablespoons water
1 tablespoon soy sauce
Japanese slaw
400g (14 oz) purple cabbage, sliced (about ¼ of a cabbage)
400g (14 oz) green cabbage, sliced (about ¼ of a cabbage)
¾ cup (9g/¼ oz) coriander (cilantro) leaves
2 green onions (scallions), thinly sliced

To make the sesame dressing, place the tahini, vinegar, water and soy in a small bowl and whisk until smooth. Set aside.

To make the Japanese slaw, place the cabbages, coriander and green onion in a large bowl and toss to combine.

Place the nori, sesame seeds and salt in a shallow dish. Press fish into nori mixture until evenly coated.

Heat a large non-stick frying pan over medium heat. Add half the oil and 2 pieces of fish to the pan. Cook for 3 minutes each side or until golden and crisp. Wipe out the pan, add the remaining oil and cook the remaining 2 pieces of fish.

To serve, divide the Japanese slaw between plates and top with the fish. Sprinkle dressing with toasted sesame seeds and drizzle over the fish. **SERVES 4**

+ *We've used snapper here, but you could use any sustainable fish that's local to you.*

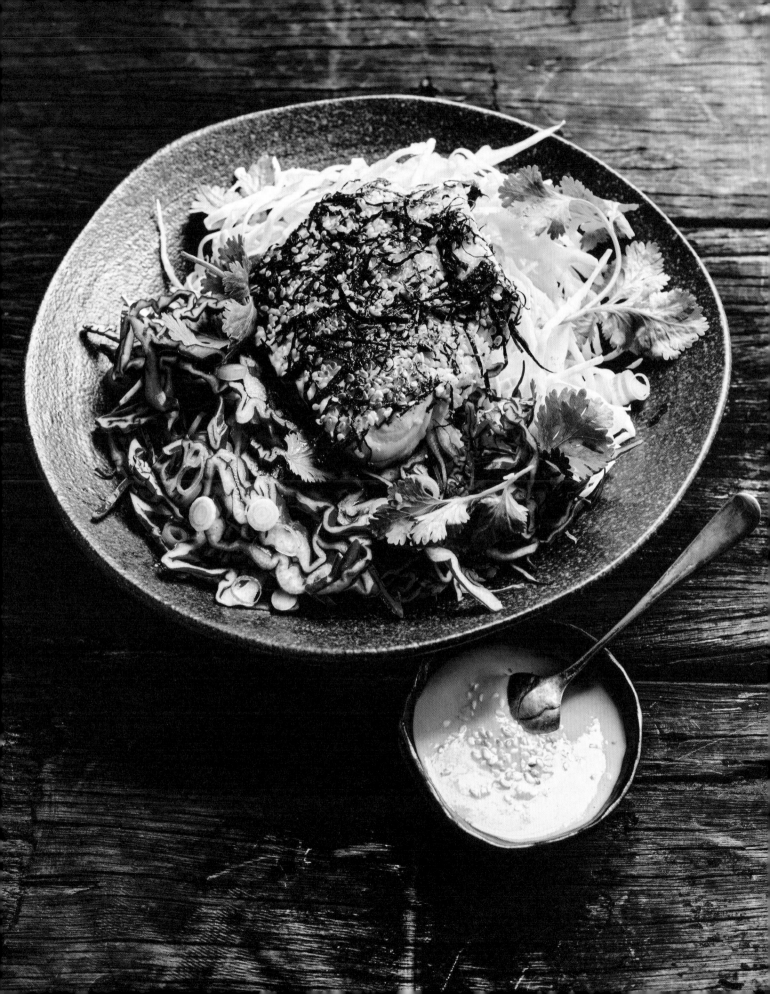

crispy NOODLE *omelettes*

150g (5¼ oz) dried rice noodles
2 cloves garlic, crushed
2 tablespoons finely grated ginger
2 tablespoons grapeseed or vegetable oil
120g (4 oz) broccolini (about 6), trimmed and halved lengthwise
8 eggs, lightly beaten
100g (3½ oz) bean sprouts, trimmed
4 green onions (scallions), sliced
½ cup (6g/¼ oz) small coriander (cilantro) sprigs
chilli sauce and kecap manis (sweet soy sauce), to serve

Place the rice noodles in a bowl and cover with boiling water. Allow to stand for 5 minutes or until soft, then drain.

Place the garlic, ginger and oil in a bowl and mix to combine. Heat a large non-stick frying pan over high heat. Add ½ the garlic mixture and cook for 1 minute. Add ½ the noodles and ½ the broccolini and cook, stirring, for 5 minutes or until the noodles are starting to crisp slightly. Add ½ the egg and swirl the pan to cover the noodles. Cook for 4 minutes or until crisp. Place ½ the bean sprouts, green onion and coriander onto the omelette and fold in half.

Remove the omelette from the pan and keep warm while you make the second omelette. Wipe the pan clean and repeat with remaining ingredients.

To serve, cut each omelette in half and divide between plates. Serve with chilli and kecap manis. **SERVES 4**

BE CREATIVE and *fill these crispy omelettes with whatever flavours* you like. Some of my favourite additions are *prawns or shredded cooked chicken.*

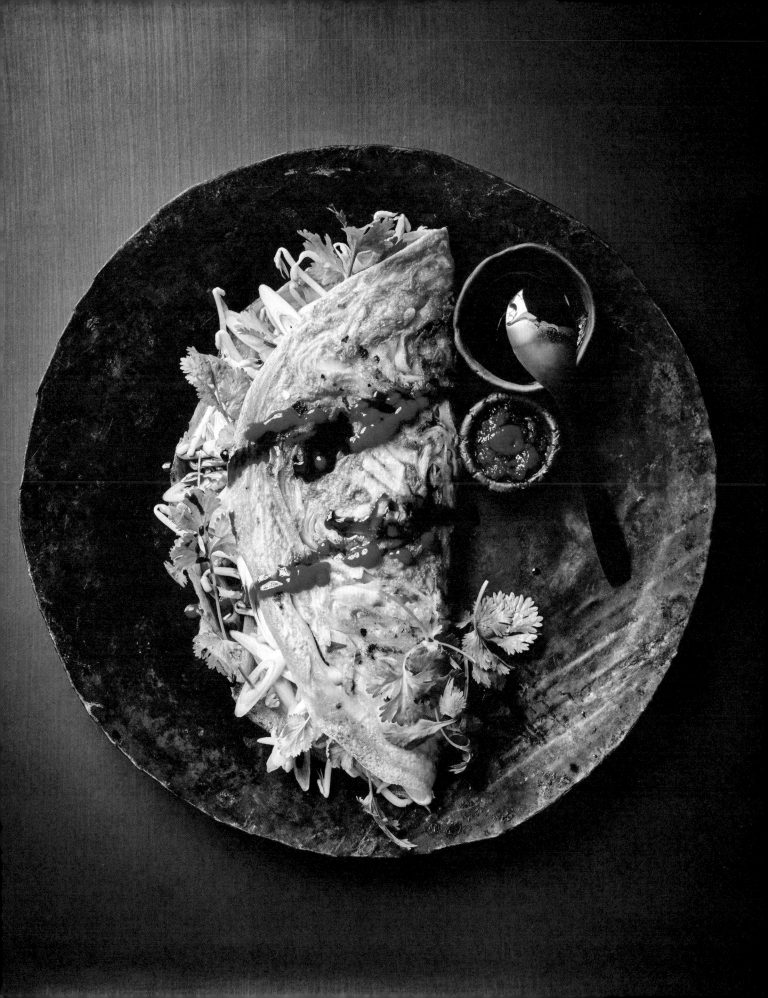

pumpkin, SAGE and *feta rolls*

1 tablespoon extra virgin olive oil
1 leek, thinly sliced
2 cups (300g/10½ oz) firmly packed grated pumpkin
2 tablespoons finely chopped sage
2 tablespoons white chia seeds
¼ cup (6g/¼ oz) chopped flat-leaf parsley leaves
⅔ cup (160g/5½ oz) fresh ricotta
120g (4¼ oz) feta
sea salt and cracked black pepper
1 x 375g (13 oz) sheet frozen spelt wholemeal (whole-wheat)
  butter puff pastry, thawed
1 egg, lightly whisked
black sesame seeds, for sprinkling
store-bought tomato chutney, to serve (optional)

Place a large deep non-stick frying pan over medium-high heat.
Add the oil and leek and cook, stirring, for 4 minutes or until soft.
  Add the pumpkin and sage and cook for 4 minutes or until soft.
Transfer to a large bowl and add the chia, parsley, ricotta, feta, salt
and pepper. Mix to combine and refrigerate until cool.
  Preheat oven to 200°C (400°F).
  Line a large baking tray with non-stick baking paper. Cut the pastry
sheet in half to make two 13.5cm x 18cm (5 inch x 7 inch) rectangles
and place on the tray. Divide pumpkin mixture between pastry pieces,
arranging it in logs along the long edges. Brush the other long edges
with egg and roll to enclose filling. Cut each roll in half to make 4 in
total. Turn rolls seam-side down on the trays. Score tops with a sharp
knife, brush with remaining egg and sprinkle with the sesame seeds.
  Bake for 20 minutes or until the pastry is puffed and golden brown.
Allow the rolls to cool on the tray for 10 minutes before serving with
tomato chutney, if you like. **MAKES 4**

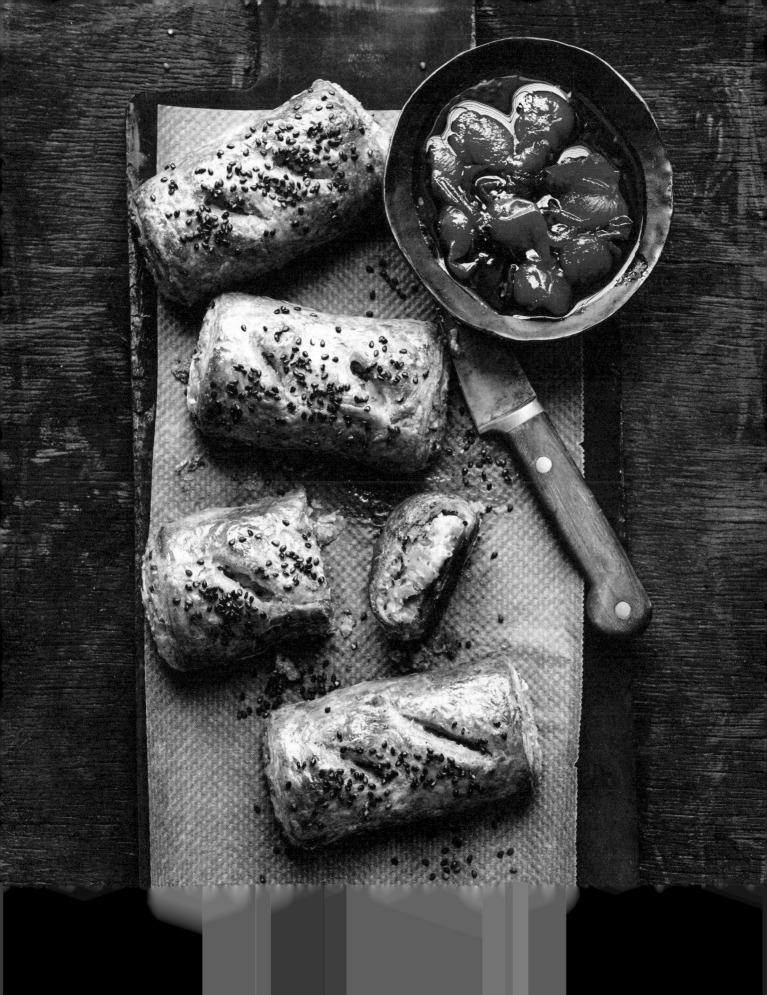

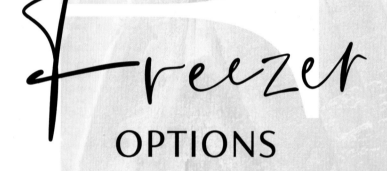

Freezer
OPTIONS

There's something deeply reassuring about a freezer stocked with NUTRITIOUS MEALS that could be *on the table in minutes*. But that doesn't mean you need to eat bolognese 24/7! These recipes offer all the *convenience of batch cooking* with built-in benefits. Think freezer-ready favourites with A LOAD OF VARIATIONS!

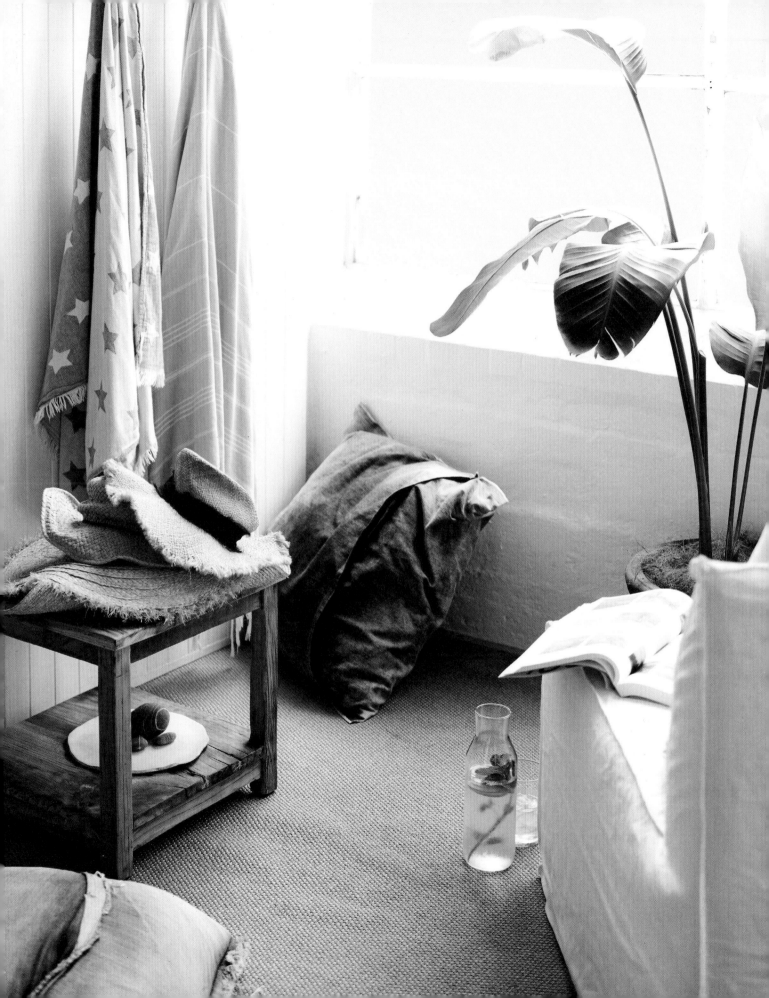

master STOCK *chicken*

6 cups (1.5 litres/50 fl oz) chicken stock
½ cup (125ml/4¼ oz) Chinese cooking wine (Shaoxing) or dry sherry
1 tablespoon soy sauce
1 tablespoon brown sugar
6–8 slices ginger
2 cloves garlic, halved
2 star anise
1 cinnamon stick
2 green onions (scallions), halved
4 strips orange peel
5 x 125g (4 oz) chicken thigh fillets, trimmed and halved

In a large saucepan over high heat, place the stock, wine, soy, sugar, ginger, garlic, star anise, cinnamon, onion and orange peel. Stir to combine. Bring to the boil, then reduce heat and simmer for 10 minutes.

Place chicken in master stock and bring to the boil. Reduce heat to low, cover and poach for 12 minutes. Remove from heat and set aside to cool in the master stock.

To freeze, remove and discard ginger, garlic, star anise, cinnamon, onion and orange peel. Refrigerate until cold, then portion into containers and transfer to freezer. Freeze for up to 3 months.

SERVES 4

The layers of FLAVOUR in this chicken soup are just perfect. *So many variations spring to mind* – GET CREATIVE!

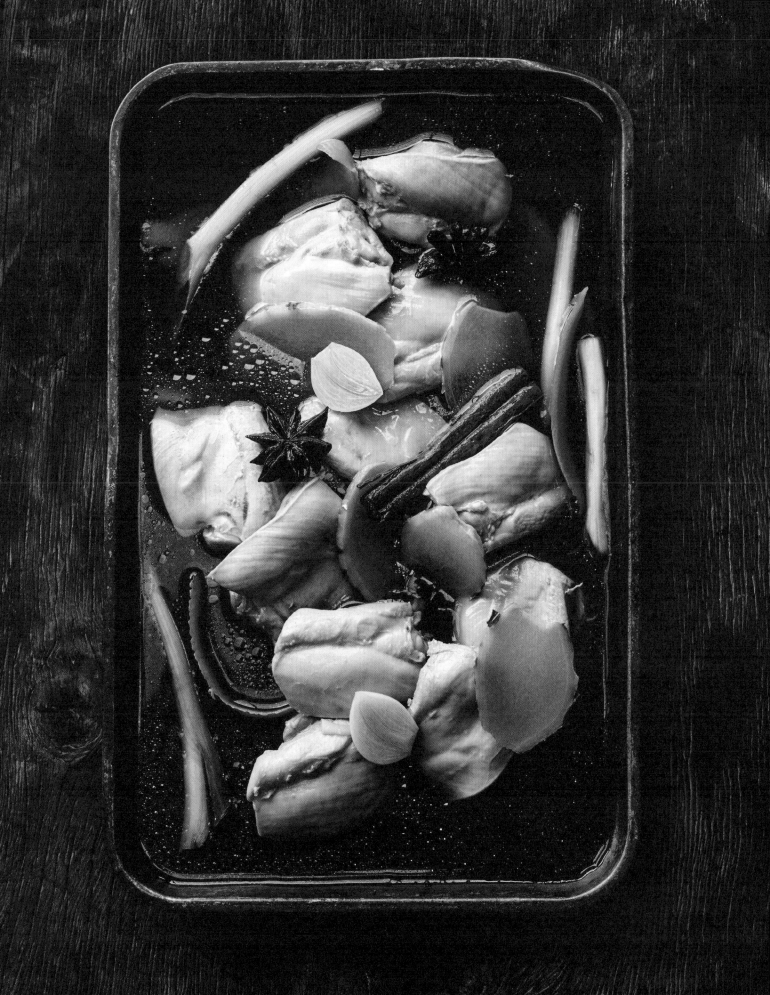

master STOCK CHICKEN
and *noodle bowl*

Heat 1 quantity of the master stock chicken (see *recipe* p148)
in a large saucepan over medium-high heat. Add 200g (7 oz)
dried rice noodles and 400g (14 oz) gai lan (Chinese broccoli)
and poach for 5 minutes. To serve, divide noodles and
broth between bowls and top with gai lan, chicken and
baby coriander (cilantro). **SERVES 4**

master STOCK CHICKEN
with *chilli greens bowl*

Heat 1 quantity of the master stock chicken (see *recipe* p148)
in a large saucepan over medium-high heat. Add 200g (7 oz)
choy sum and 200g (7 oz) pak choy and poach for 5 minutes
or until cooked. To serve, divide broth, choy sum, pak choy
and chicken between bowls and top with coriander (cilantro)
sprigs and fried chilli and ginger. **SERVES 4**

pork AND fennel *meatballs*

1 cup (70g/2½ oz) wholemeal (whole-wheat) fresh breadcrumbs
¼ cup (60ml/2 fl oz) milk
2 teaspoons fennel seeds, plus ¼ teaspoon extra
1 teaspoon sea salt flakes
550g (1 lb 2 oz) pork mince[+]
2 teaspoons honey
¼ cup (20g/¾ oz) finely chopped flat-leaf parsley leaves
2 tablespoons extra virgin olive oil
2 sprigs rosemary

In a small bowl, place breadcrumbs and milk. Mix to combine and set aside for 2 minutes to soak.

Place fennel and salt in a mortar and pestle and gently crush.

In a large bowl, place pork, breadcrumb mixture, fennel salt, honey and parsley and mix to combine. Roll heaped tablespoonfuls of mince mixture into balls.

Heat a large non-stick frying pan over medium-high heat. Add the oil, rosemary and extra fennel and cook for 2 minutes or until fragrant. Add the meatballs and cook, turning occasionally, for 8–10 minutes or until browned all over and cooked through.

To freeze, allow meatballs to cool, then layer between non-stick baking paper in an airtight container. Freeze for up to 3 months.

SERVES 4

+ *If you prefer, you could swap the pork mince for chicken mince.*

A GREAT MEATBALL should be well flavoured enough to *fit any occasion at a moment's notice* – from a HEARTY PASTA to a drinks platter for when friends drop by.

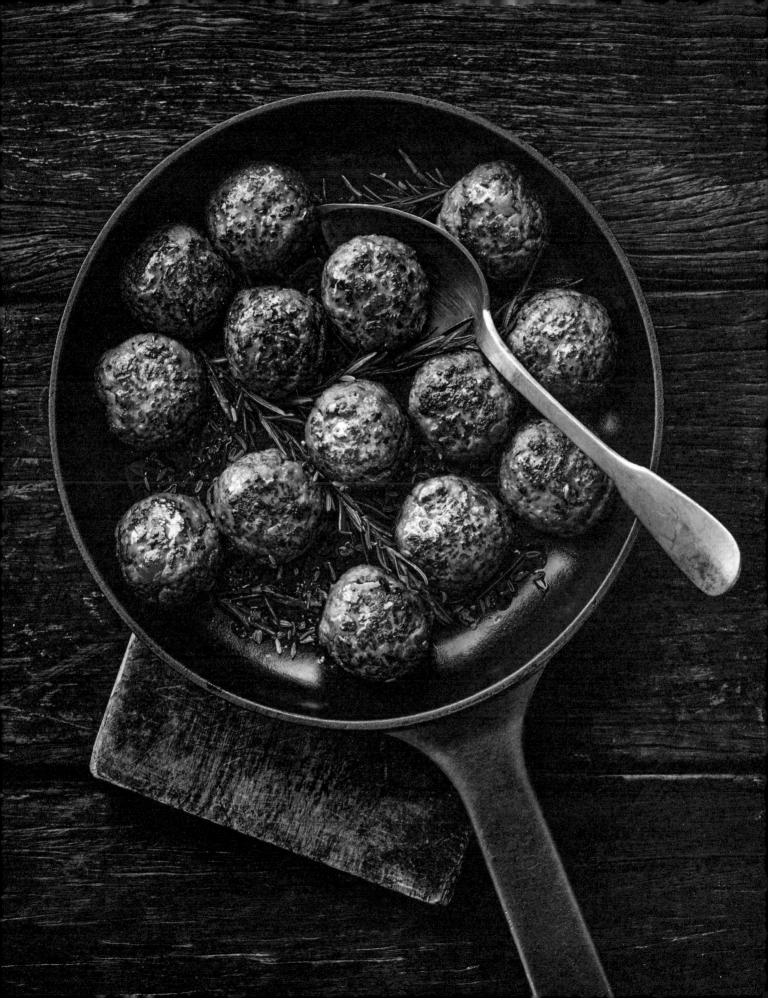

pork AND FENNEL MEATBALLS
ploughman's *mezze board*

Heat 1 quantity of the pork and fennel meatballs (see *recipe* p152) in a non-stick frying pan over medium-high heat until warm. To serve, place the meatballs on a platter with freshly sliced sourdough or wholemeal (whole-wheat) bread, char-grilled zucchini (courgette) slices, charred radicchio, green olives, sliced cornichons and baby spinach leaves. **SERVES 4**

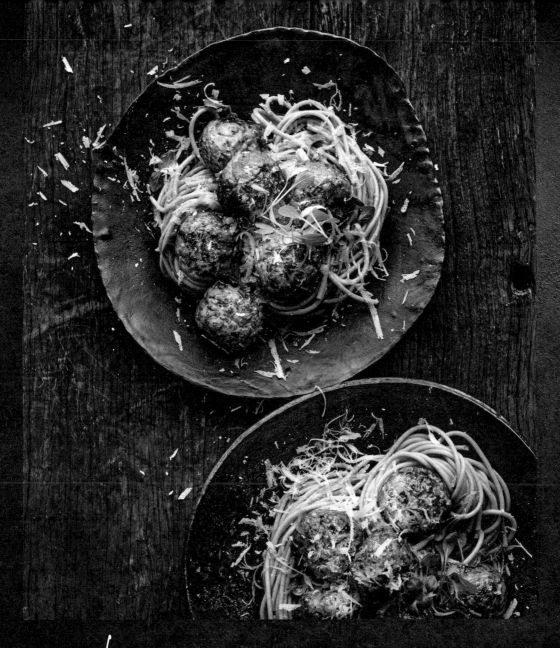

pork AND FENNEL MEATBALLS with
whole-wheat pasta, parmesan and lemon

Heat 1 quantity of the pork and fennel meatballs (see *recipe* p152) in a non-stick frying pan over medium-high heat until warm. Cook 400g (14 oz) dried wholemeal (whole-wheat) spaghetti in a large saucepan of boiling salted water for 8 minutes or until al dente. Drain and add 1 tablespoon of finely grated lemon rind to the pasta and mix to combine. To serve, divide pasta between bowls and top with the pork and fennel meatballs, finely grated parmesan, baby basil, salt and pepper. **SERVES 4**

green
MINESTRONE *soup*

1 tablespoon extra virgin olive oil
1 leek, trimmed and sliced
6 cups (1.5 litres/50 fl oz) chicken or vegetable stock
½ cup (110g/3¾ oz) freekeh, rinsed and drained
2 small zucchini (courgettes), grated
250g (8¾ oz) broccoli, cut into small florets
150g (5 oz) green beans, trimmed and chopped
1 cup (140g/4¼ oz) frozen shelled edamame beans
1 tablespoon finely grated lemon rind
¼ cup (6g/¼ oz) flat-leaf parsley leaves
¼ cup (4g/¼ oz) mint leaves
sea salt and cracked black pepper
finely grated parmesan, to serve

Heat a large saucepan over medium-high heat. Add oil and leek
and cook for 5 minutes. Add stock and freekeh and bring to the boil.
Reduce heat to a simmer, cover and cook for 30 minutes.
   Add zucchini, broccoli, green beans and edamame and cook,
uncovered, for 10 minutes.
   Stir through lemon rind, parsley, mint and salt and pepper.
Serve scattered with parmesan.
   To freeze, allow to cool, divide between airtight containers and
freeze for up to 3 months. **SERVES 4**

**Minestrone just got a FRESHEN UP with *all my
favourite greens and zesty lemon and herbs*. A perfect
soup to have on STAND-BY in the freezer.**

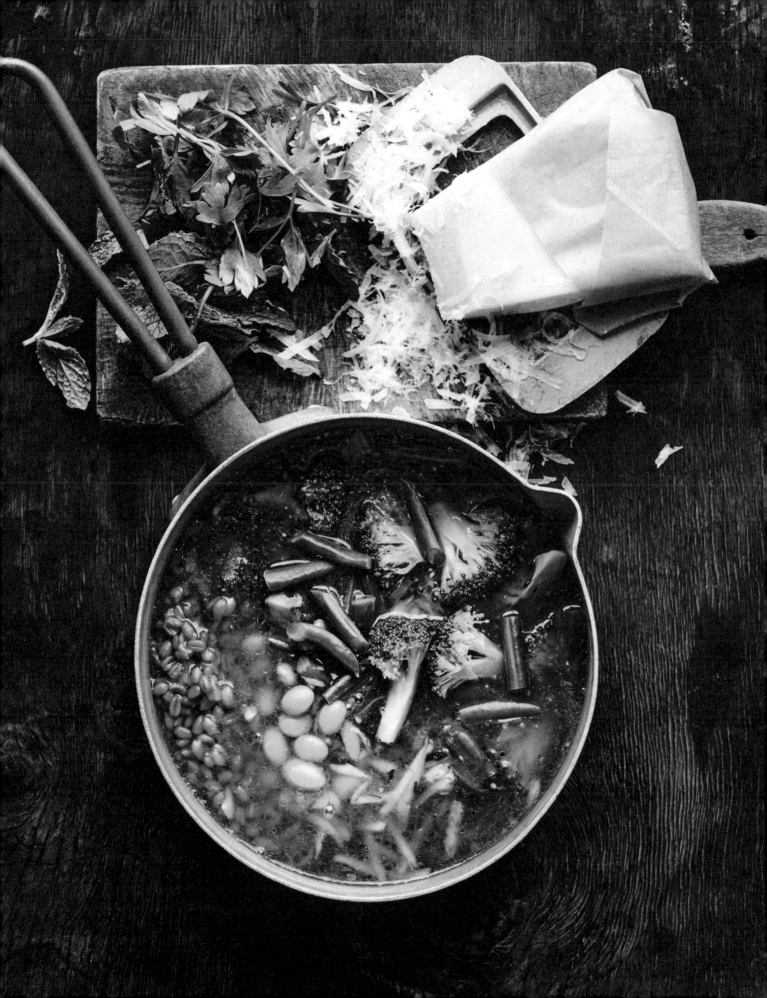

green MINESTRONE SOUP
with *mint pesto*

Heat 1 quantity of the green minestrone soup (see *recipe* p156)
in a large saucepan over medium-high heat. To make the mint
pesto, place ⅓ cup (5g/¼ oz) roughly chopped mint, ¼ cup
(20g/¾ oz) finely grated parmesan, 2 tablespoons toasted
and roughly chopped pine nuts, 1 teaspoon finely grated
lemon rind, ¼ cup (60ml/2 fl oz) extra virgin olive oil, salt and
pepper in a medium bowl and mix to combine. To serve, divide
minestrone between bowls and top with minted pesto. **SERVES 4**

green MINESTRONE SOUP
with *maple pancetta*

Heat 1 quantity of the green minestrone soup (see *recipe* p156) in a large saucepan over medium-high heat. To make the maple pancetta, heat the grill to high. Brush one side of 12 thin slices of pancetta with maple syrup and grill until crisp. To serve, divide the green minestrone soup between bowls and top with maple pancetta and finely grated parmesan. **SERVES 4**

asian SPICED
lemongrass *pork*

6 thin slices of ginger

2 cloves garlic, roughly chopped

2 stalks lemongrass, trimmed and chopped

2 large red chillies, seeds removed and chopped, plus extra sliced
  chilli to serve

½ red onion, chopped

4 kaffir lime leaves, finely shredded, plus extra finely shredded
  leaves, to serve

1 tablespoon extra virgin olive oil

500g (1 lb 1 oz) pork mince[+]

finely shredded green onion (scallion), to serve

sauce

2 tablespoons rice wine vinegar

1 tablespoon fish sauce

1 tablespoon brown sugar

Combine ginger, garlic, lemongrass, chilli, red onion and kaffir lime
leaves in a small food processor and process to form a fine mixture.

Heat a large non-stick frying pan over medium-high heat. Add the
oil and the ginger mixture and cook for 5 minutes or until fragrant.

Add the pork mince to the ginger mixture and cook, breaking up
mince with a wooden spoon, for 8 minutes or until golden.

To make the sauce, in a small bowl add the vinegar, fish sauce and
sugar and mix to combine. Add to the mince mixture and stir well to
ensure the sugar dissolves.

Serve topped with green onion, extra chilli and kaffir lime leaves.

To freeze, allow to cool before placing in an airtight container in the
freezer. Freeze for up to 3 months. **SERVES 4**

+ *If you prefer, you could swap the pork mince for chicken mince.*

There's something so right about having such
a complete FLAVOURED BASE in the freezer –
it makes your defrost dinner options not just
SUPER EASY but exciting too!

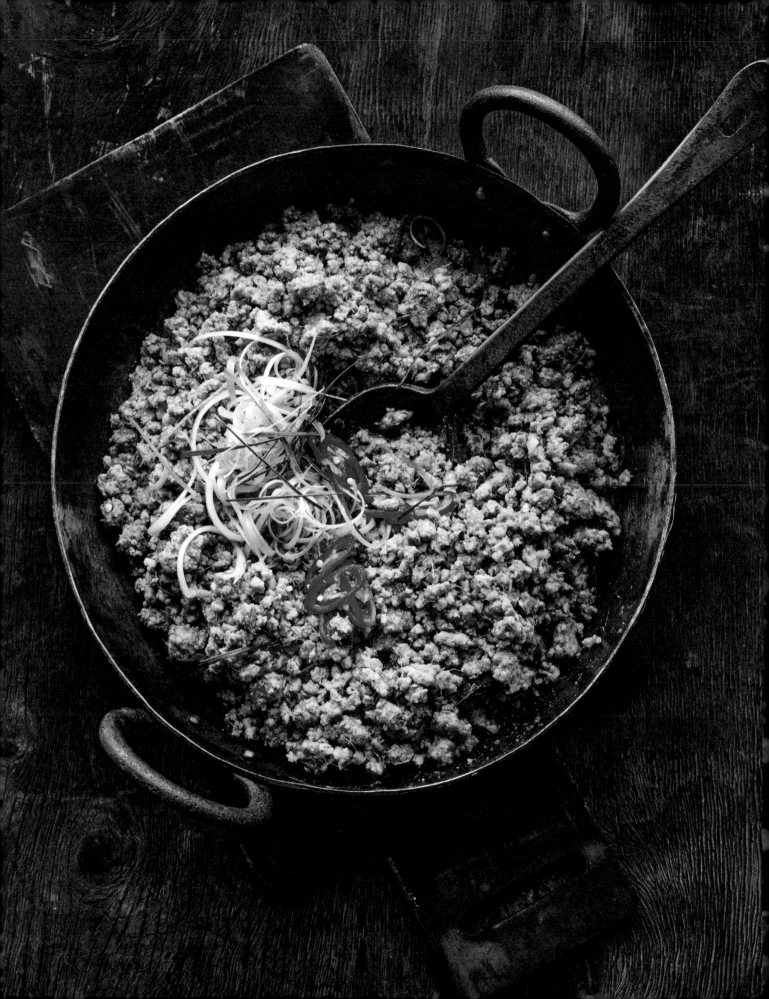

asian SPICED LEMONGRASS PORK
with *noodles and beans*

Heat 1 quantity Asian spiced lemongrass pork (see *recipe* p160) in a large non-stick frying pan over medium-high heat. In a large bowl, place 200g (7 oz) dried rice noodles and add boiling water. Cook following the packet instructions. To serve, divide noodles, 350g (12 oz) halved and blanched green beans and the Asian spiced lemongrass pork between bowls. Top with mint, Thai basil, thinly sliced green chilli and lime wedges. **SERVES 4**

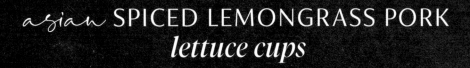

asian SPICED LEMONGRASS PORK
lettuce cups

Heat 1 quantity Asian spiced lemongrass pork (see *recipe*
p160) in a large non-stick frying pan over medium-high heat.
Place 3 shredded cucumbers in a bowl with ⅔ cup
(8g/¼ oz) coriander (cilantro) leaves and ⅔ cup (10g/¼ oz)
mint leaves. Mix to combine. To serve, divide the Asian spiced
lemongrass pork between 8–12 butter lettuce leaves and
top with the cucumber salad and thinly sliced green chilli.
Serve with lime wedges. **SERVES 4**

cheat's ROAST
pumpkin *soup*

1.8kg (4 lb) butternut pumpkin, halved and seeds removed
2 brown onions, halved with skin on
1 bulb garlic
¼ cup (60ml/2 fl oz) extra virgin olive oil
sea salt and cracked black pepper
4 cups (1 litre/34 fl oz) chicken or vegetable stock
1 cup (250ml/8½ fl oz) water
⅓ cup (80ml/2¾ fl oz) single (pouring) cream
2 teaspoons Dijon mustard

Preheat oven to 220°C (425°F).

Place the pumpkin and onion, cut-side up, and the garlic on a large oven tray lined with non-stick baking paper. Drizzle with the oil and sprinkle with salt and pepper. Cover with a sheet of non-stick baking paper and then cover with aluminium foil to seal.

Bake for 45 minutes, then remove the foil and baking paper. Bake for a further 20 minutes or until the onion is caramelised and pumpkin is soft. Set aside until cool enough to handle. Scoop out the flesh of the pumpkin into a large saucepan. Remove the onion and garlic from their skins and add to the saucepan.

Add the stock and water. Using a hand-held blender, blend the soup until smooth. Place the soup over high heat and bring to the boil to heat through.

Combine cream and Dijon in a small bowl. Serve soup with a sprinkle of pepper and drizzled with the Dijon cream.

To freeze, omit adding the Dijon cream. Allow soup to cool then freeze in airtight containers for up to 3 months. **SERVES 4**

My classic NO PEEL pumpkin soup has become *lots of people's go-to recipe*, so I've created FLAVOUR OPTIONS for you to *take a fave to the next level.*

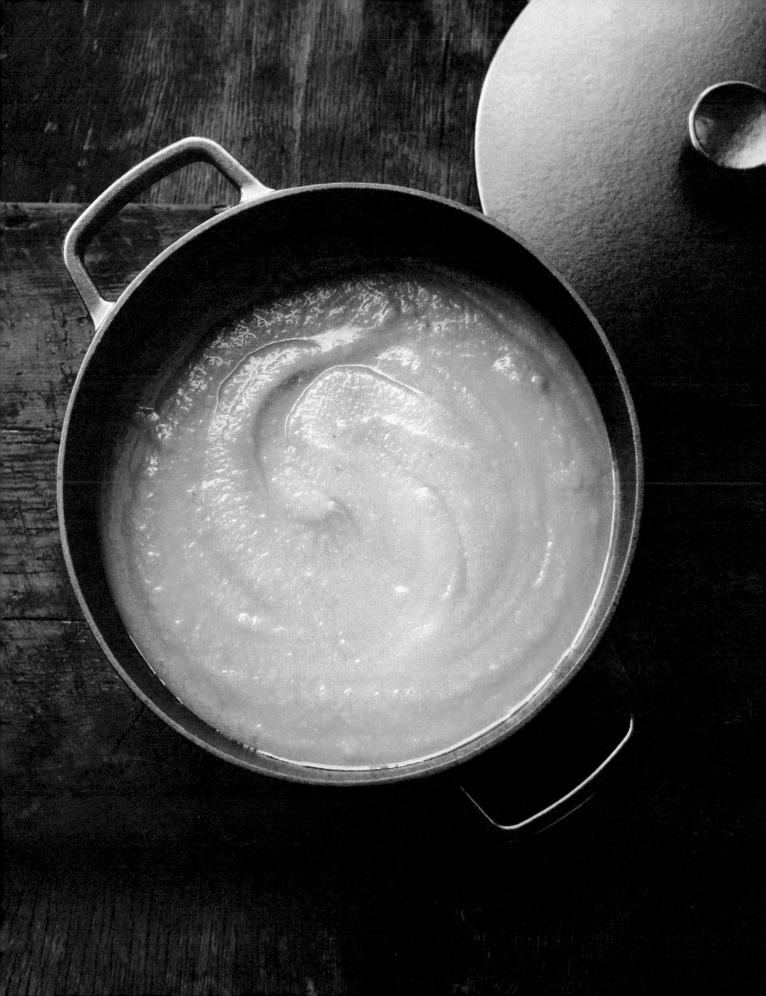

spiced RED CURRY
pumpkin soup

Heat a large saucepan over medium-high heat and
cook 2 tablespoons of red curry paste for 2 minutes or until
fragrant. Add ½ cup (125ml/4¼ oz) coconut cream and stir
to combine. Add 1 quantity of the cheat's roast pumpkin
soup (see *recipe* p164) and heat for 4–5 minutes, stirring
occasionally, until warm. To serve, divide soup between bowls
and swirl with extra coconut cream. Top with coriander
(cilantro) leaves and thinly sliced red and green chilli. **SERVES 4**

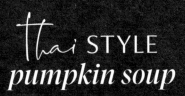

thai STYLE
pumpkin soup

Heat 1 quantity of the cheat's roast pumpkin soup (see *recipe* p164) in a large saucepan over medium-high heat. Add 400g (14 oz) thinly sliced chicken breast, along with 2 teaspoons fish sauce and 1½ tablespoons lime juice. Cook, stirring, for 2 minutes or until chicken is cooked through. Add ¼ cup (3g/¼ oz) chopped coriander (cilantro) leaves and stir to combine. Divide soup between bowls and serve with thinly sliced green chilli, purple shiso leaves and lime cheeks. **SERVES 4**

black BEAN *bolognese*

1 tablespoon extra virgin olive oil
1 brown onion, chopped
1 clove garlic, crushed
250g (9 oz) beef mince
1 x 400g (14 oz) can cherry tomatoes
1 x 400g (14 oz) can black beans, rinsed and drained
½ cup (125ml/4¼ fl oz) tomato puree (passata)
½ cup (125ml/4¼ fl oz) beef stock
sea salt and cracked black pepper

Heat a large deep frying pan over medium heat. Add the oil, onion and garlic. Cook for 5 minutes or until onion is just soft. Add the mince and cook, stirring, for about 5 minutes or until browned.

Add the tomatoes, beans, tomato puree, stock, salt and pepper and simmer, stirring occasionally, for 20 minutes or until thickened.

To freeze, allow to cool before placing in an airtight container and freeze for up to 3 months. SERVES 4

Sure there's nothing new about having bolognese in the freezer, but when you add SUPER-CHARGED black beans and *pops of sweet cherry tomatoes*, you get a whole new level of DELICIOUSNESS.

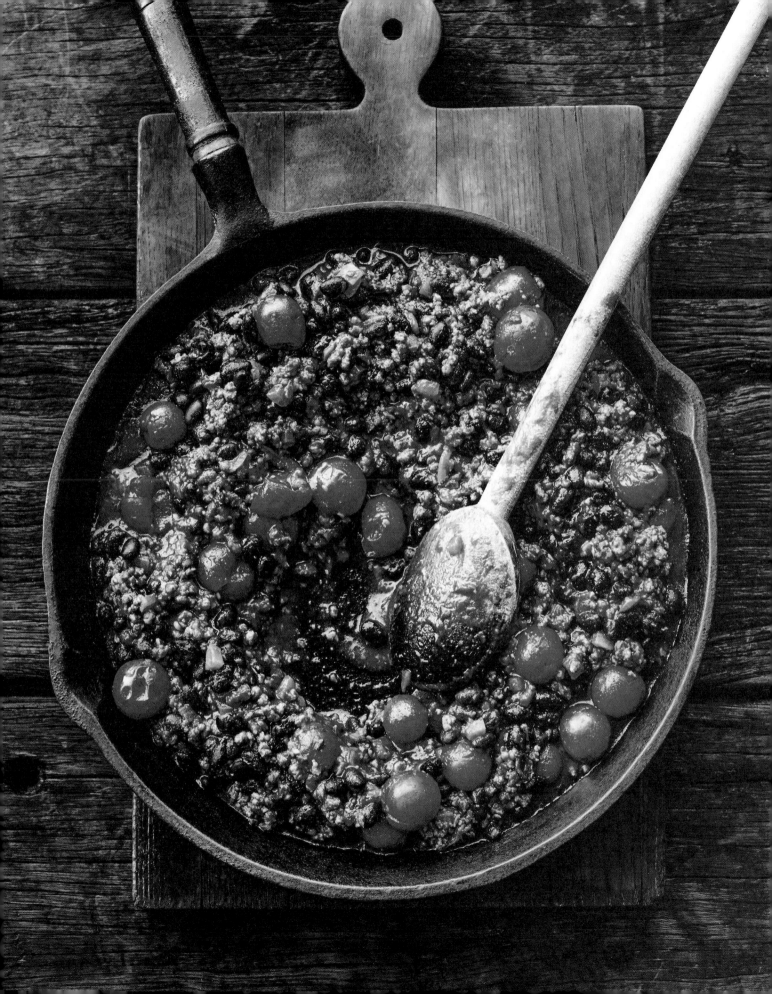

black BEAN BOLOGNESE
with *vegetable spaghetti*

Warm 1 quantity of the black bean bolognese (see *recipe* p168) in a large deep frying pan over medium heat. Cook 200g (7 oz) wholemeal (whole-wheat) spaghetti in a large saucepan of salted boiling water for 8 minutes or until al dente. Drain and set aside. Using a julienne peeler, shred 2 x 200g (7 oz) zucchini (courgettes) and 2 x 200g (7 oz) carrots. To serve, divide the zucchini, carrot and pasta between bowls and top with the black bean bolognese, basil leaves and finely grated parmesan. **SERVES 4**

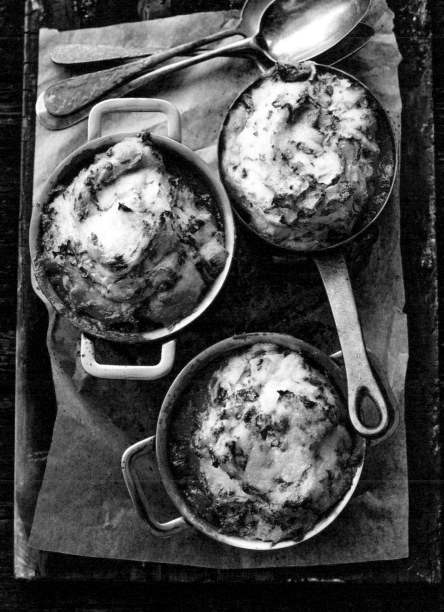

black BEAN BOLOGNESE PIE
with *parsnip, celeriac and kale*

Heat a frying pan over medium heat. Add 1 tablespoon extra
virgin olive oil and 1 thinly sliced leek. Cook, stirring, for
5 minutes until softened. Add 250g (9 oz) each of peeled and
chopped parsnip and celeriac. Cook for 1 minute. Add ½ cup
(125ml/4¼ fl oz) milk. Cover and cook for 30 minutes until soft.
Blend or mash until smooth. Stir in ¾ cup (25g/¾ oz) shredded
kale leaves (stems removed). Preheat oven to 220°C (425°F).
Divide 1 quantity of reheated black bean bolognese (see *recipe*
p168) between 4 x 1½ cup (375ml/12½ fl oz) capacity pie dishes.
Top with the mash. Bake for 15 minutes until browned. **SERVES 4**

171

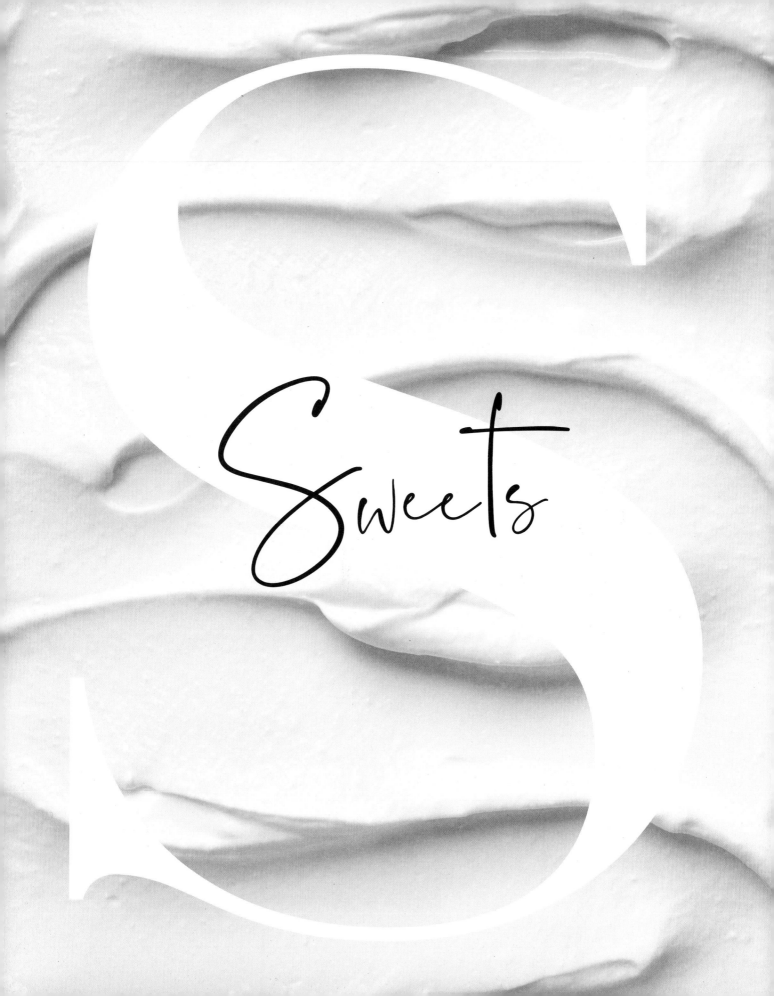

Sweets

In recent years, the way I approach sweet treats and desserts *has evolved*. Coming up with clever and delicious ways to *reduce the* ADDED SUGAR but not the SATISFACTION has been an exciting challenge. These sweets will trigger the *nostalgic delight* of your favourite cheesecakes, pies and crumbles but with A LITTLE MORE BALANCE.

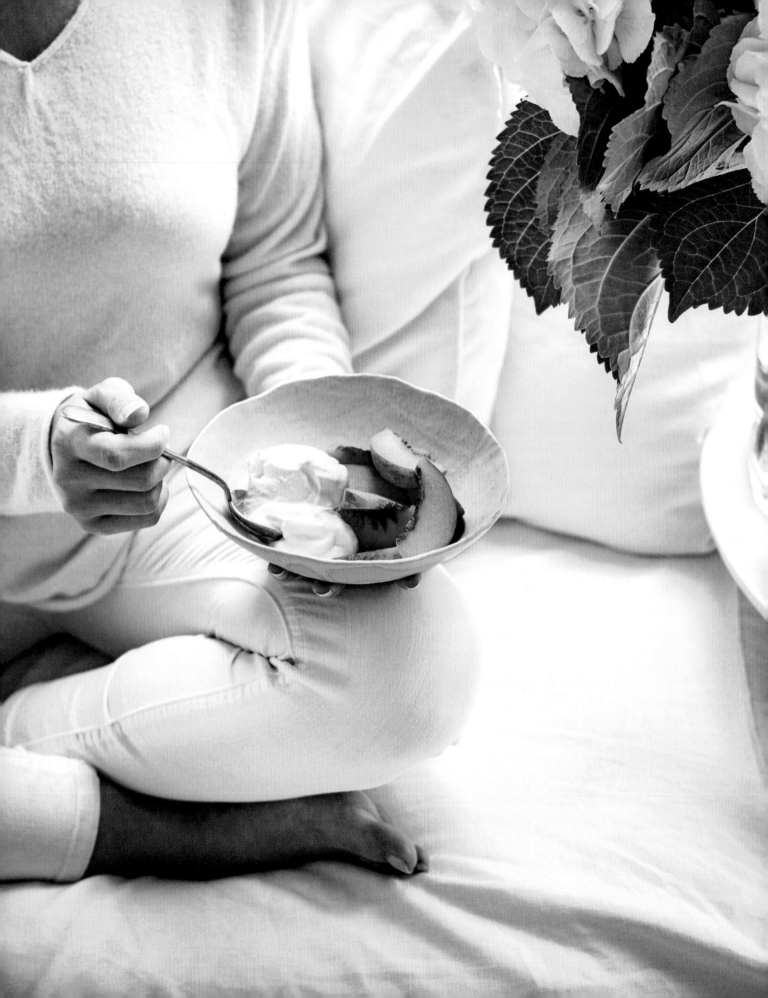

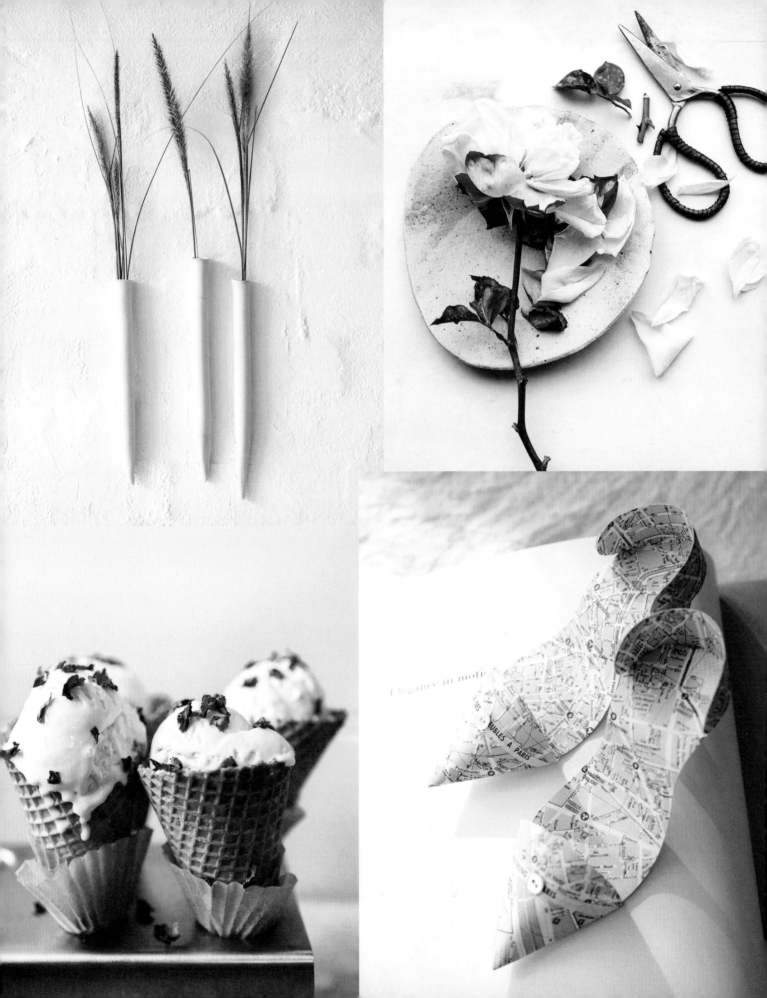

summer FRUITS with *toasted honey marshmallow*

4–5 mixed seasonal stone fruits
¼ cup (55g/2oz) raw caster (superfine) sugar
2 cups (250g/8¾ oz) frozen raspberries
honey marshmallow
2 egg whites
1 teaspoon vanilla bean paste
1 tablespoon honey

Preheat oven to 180°C (350°F).

Cut stone fruits in half, remove and discard stones and place cut-side up on a baking tray lined with non-stick baking paper. Sprinkle the fruit with 1 tablespoon of the sugar.

Toss raspberries and remaining sugar together in a bowl and place around stone fruit on baking tray. Bake for 10 minutes, then remove from the oven and set aside.

Increase the oven temperature to 220°C (425°C).

Using a stand mixer or handheld mixer, whisk egg whites and vanilla until soft peaks form. Slowly add honey and continue to whisk until thick and glossy. Place spoonfuls of the honey marshmallow on top of the stone fruit. Return to the oven and bake for 3 minutes or until golden and toasted. **SERVES 4**

This super-easy TRAY BAKE dessert celebrates *my favourite summer fruits.* All the flavours work in harmony – from the tang of the raspberry pan sauce to the SWEET CLOUD of *honeyed marshmallow.*

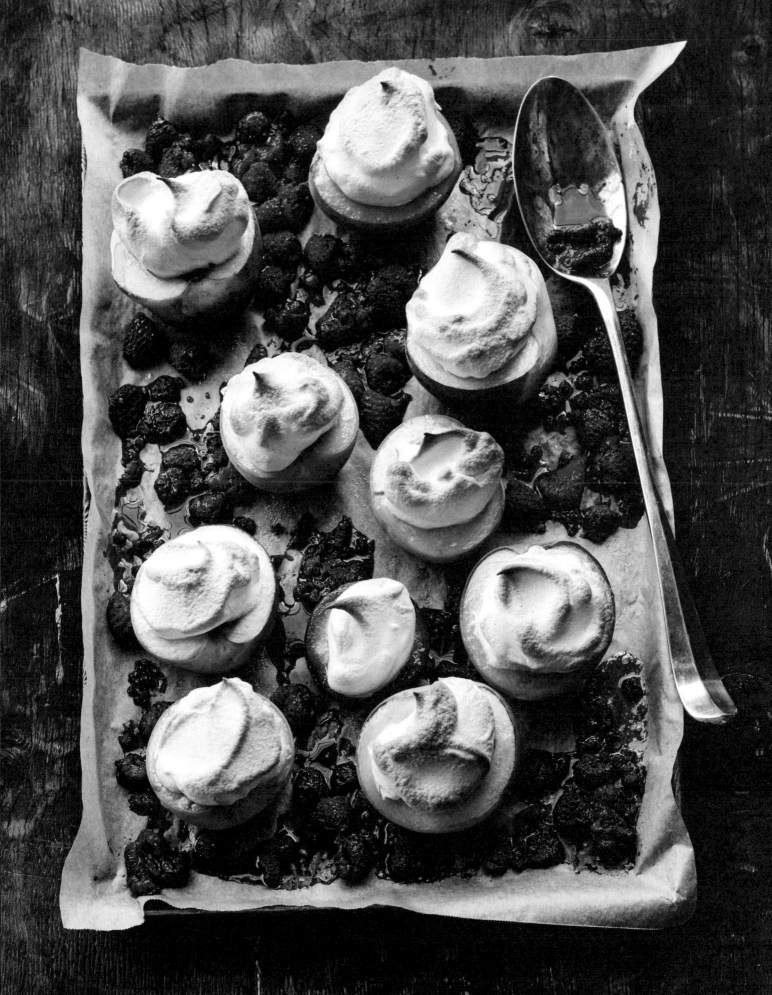

mango and COCONUT SNOW

toasted flaked coconut, to serve
coconut snow
½ cup (125ml/4½ fl oz) boiling water
½ cup (110g/4 oz) raw caster (superfine) sugar
2 cups (500ml/17 fl oz) coconut milk
1 teaspoon vanilla extract
mango snow
⅓ cup (80ml/2¾ fl oz) boiling water
¼ cup (55g/2 oz) raw caster (superfine) sugar
1½ cups (375ml/12½ fl oz) fresh mango puree (about 3 mangoes)
2 tablespoons lime juice
1 teaspoon grated lime rind

To make the coconut snow, place the water and sugar in a heatproof bowl and stir to dissolve. Add the coconut milk and vanilla and stir to combine. Pour into a large flat metal dish and freeze for 2 hours.

To make the mango snow, place the water and sugar in a heatproof bowl and stir to dissolve. Add the mango, lime juice and rind, and stir to combine. Pour into a large flat metal dish and freeze for 2 hours.

Rake each mixture with a fork then return to the freezer for 1 hour or until firm.

To serve, rake the mixtures again and spoon into bowls. Sprinkle with toasted coconut flakes. **SERVES 4–6**

This is my kind of dessert. DELICATE tropical snow that's on the *right side of sweetness.* It's such a *refreshing treat.* Serve it in coconut halves for a super-fun ISLAND VIBE.

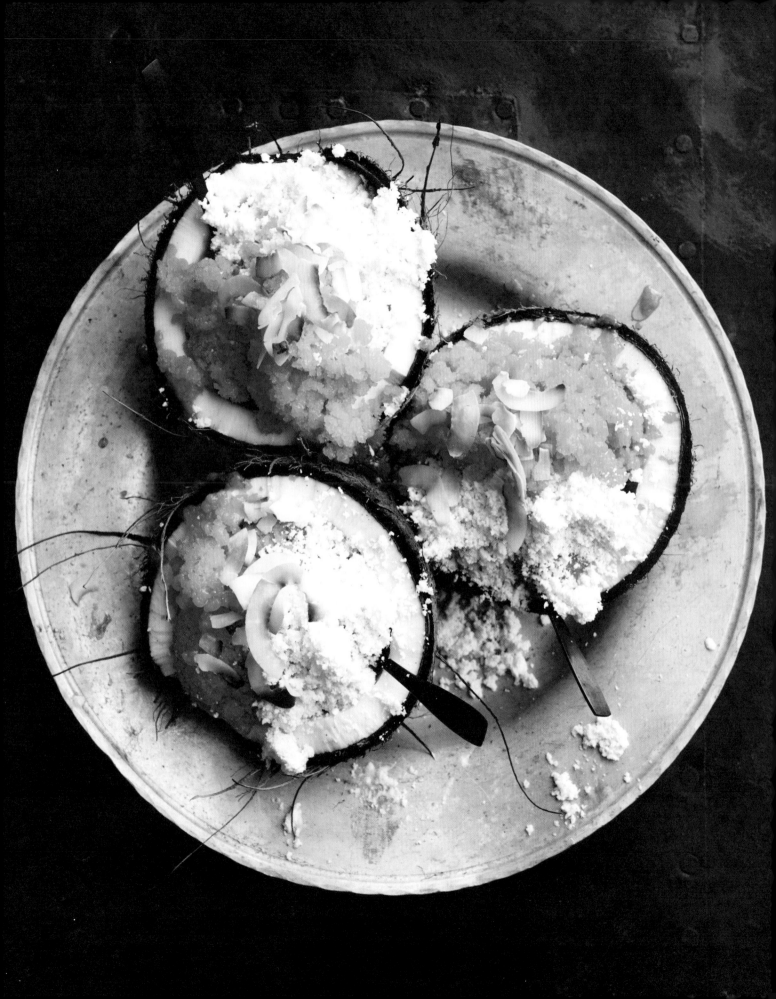

passionfruit, CHIA and coconut slice

½ cup (60g/2 oz) almond meal (ground almonds)
½ cup (40g/1½ oz) desiccated coconut
⅓ cup (80g/2¾ oz) almond butter
2 tablespoons raw caster (superfine) sugar
2 tablespoons pure maple syrup
passionfruit chia filling
1½ cups (360g/12½ oz) fresh passionfruit pulp
¼ cup (60ml/2 fl oz) pure maple syrup
2 tablespoons white chia seeds
coconut topping
1½ cups (115g/4 oz) shredded coconut
2 egg whites
2 tablespoons raw caster (superfine) sugar

Preheat oven to 160°C (325°F).

To make the passionfruit chia filling, place the passionfruit and maple into a saucepan over medium heat. Bring to a rapid simmer and simmer for 8–10 minutes or until the mixture has thickened slightly. Remove from heat and stir through the chia seeds and set aside for 20 minutes.

To make the base, line a 20cm (8 inch) square cake tin with non-stick baking paper. Mix together the almond meal, coconut, almond butter, sugar and maple. Press into the base of the tin and bake for 15 minutes or until golden. Set aside for 15 minutes to cool.

While the base is cooling, make the coconut topping. Combine the coconut, egg whites and sugar.

Pour the passionfruit filling over the base and top with the coconut topping. Bake for 20 minutes or until lightly golden brown. Refrigerate for 2–3 hours or until cold. To serve, cut into slices. **MAKES 12 SQUARES**

For me the combination of passionfruit and coconut TASTES LIKE SUMMER. I've captured the essence of this in a *perfectly portable slice.*

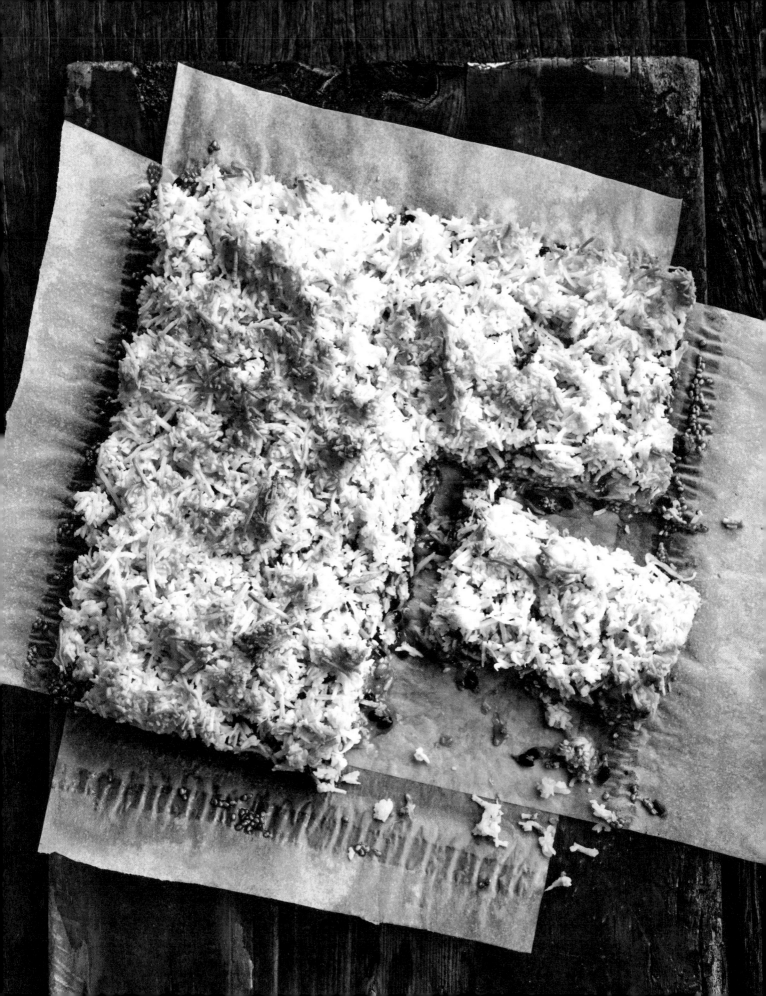

coconut ICE-CREAM and *miso caramel swirl*

3 x 400g (14 oz) cans coconut cream[+]
1 cup (250ml/8½ fl oz) light agave syrup
2 teaspoons vanilla extract
½ teaspoon xanthan gum
miso caramel
1½ tablespoons white miso paste (shiro)
½ cup (125ml/4¼ fl oz) pure maple syrup
1 teaspoon vanilla extract

Place a 20cm (8 inch) square metal tin in the freezer.

Place coconut cream, agave and vanilla in the bowl of an electric mixer and freeze for 30 minutes. Whip the coconut mixture, then with motor running, sieve over the xanthan gum and whip until thick and creamy. Pour into the chilled tin and freeze for 6 hours or overnight.

To make the miso caramel, place miso, maple and vanilla in a saucepan over low heat. Cook, stirring occasionally, until smooth and thickened slightly. Allow to cool.

Remove ice-cream from freezer about 10 minutes before serving. To serve, divide coconut ice-cream between bowls and top with the miso caramel. **SERVES 8**
+ *We found that good-quality thick and creamy coconut cream works best for this recipe.*

The umami of miso gives this updated SALTED CARAMEL a new depth of flavour. It's a *stunning partner for the rich creamy coconut ice-cream.*

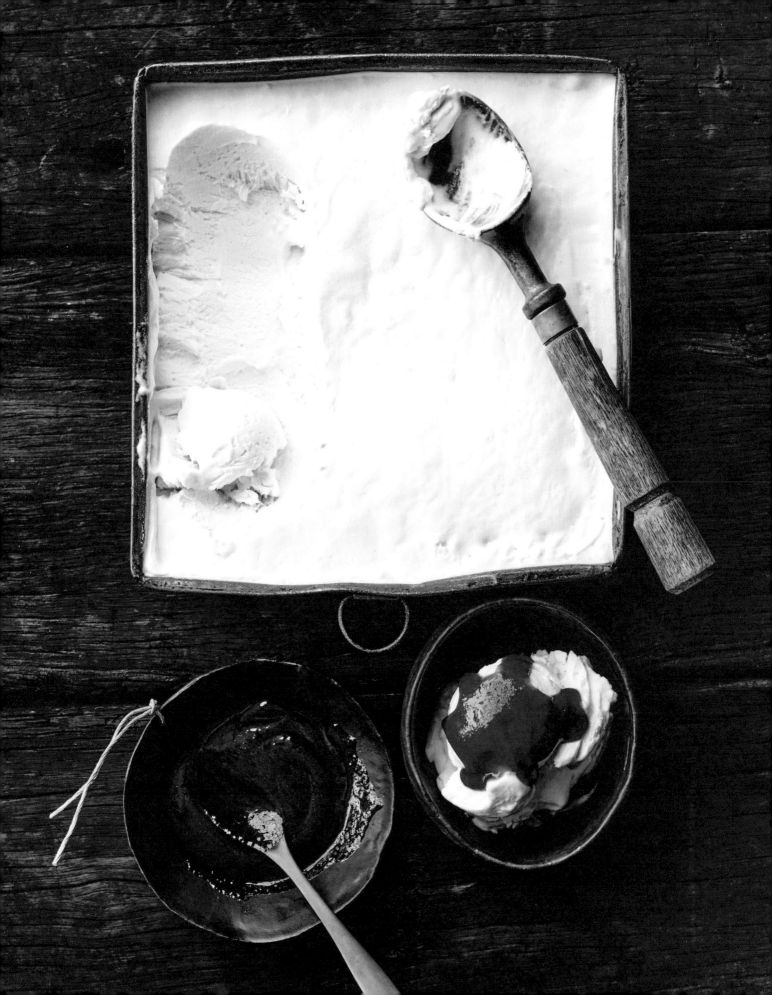

grilled VANILLA PEACHES
with almond crunch

4 peaches, halved and stones removed
2 teaspoons vanilla bean paste
coconut or vanilla ice-cream, to serve (optional)
almond crunch
½ cup (60g/2 oz) almond meal (ground almonds)
¼ cup (50g/1¾ oz) flaked almonds
¼ cup (55g/2 oz) raw caster (superfine) sugar
2 teaspoons water
sea salt flakes

Preheat oven to 160°C (325°F).

To make the almond crunch, place the almond meal, almonds, sugar and water into a bowl and mix to combine. Spoon onto a baking tray lined with non-stick baking paper and flatten slightly. Sprinkle with a little sea salt. Bake for 20 minutes or until golden. Allow to cool on the tray.

To grill the peaches, preheat a barbecue char-grill or char-grill pan to high. Brush the cut side of each peach with vanilla. Cook for 1–2 minutes or until lightly charred.

To serve, place peaches on serving plates and top with the almond crunch. Serve with a scoop of ice-cream if desired. **SERVES 4**

A flash on the char-grill and *a brush of vanilla* brings out the NATURAL SWEETNESS of summer stone fruits. Add layers of texture with *crunchy almond crumble* and velvety ice-cream. HEAVEN!

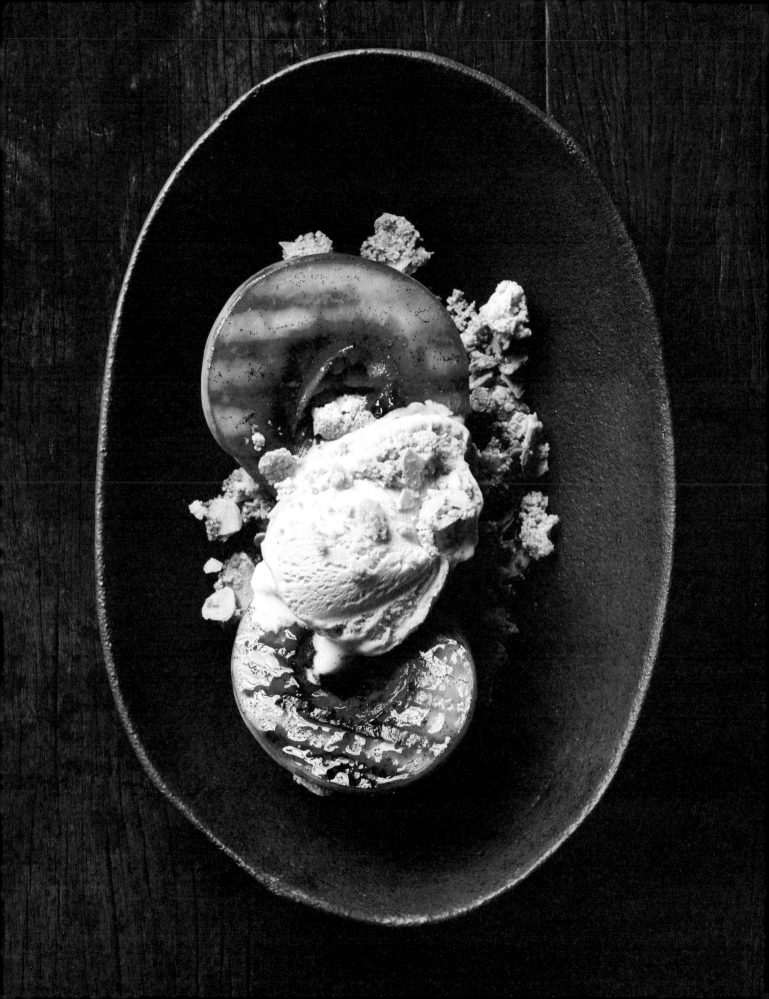

aperol SPRITZ
granita

1 cup (250ml/8½ fl oz) Aperol
1 cup (250ml/8½ fl oz) prosecco
¾ cup (180ml/6 fl oz) light agave syrup
1 cup (250ml/8½ fl oz) soda water
1½ cups (375ml/12½ fl oz) orange juice
1 orange, sliced, to serve

Place the Aperol, prosecco, agave, soda water and orange juice into a bowl and mix to combine. Pour mixture into a metal container and freeze for 3 hours or overnight until just set.

To serve, rake the granita with a fork. Serve in glasses with slices of orange. **SERVES 4**

Here's another excuse to indulge in everyone's *favourite summer drink.* I've SPRITZED UP the flavours to create a *refreshingly icy Aperol treat.*

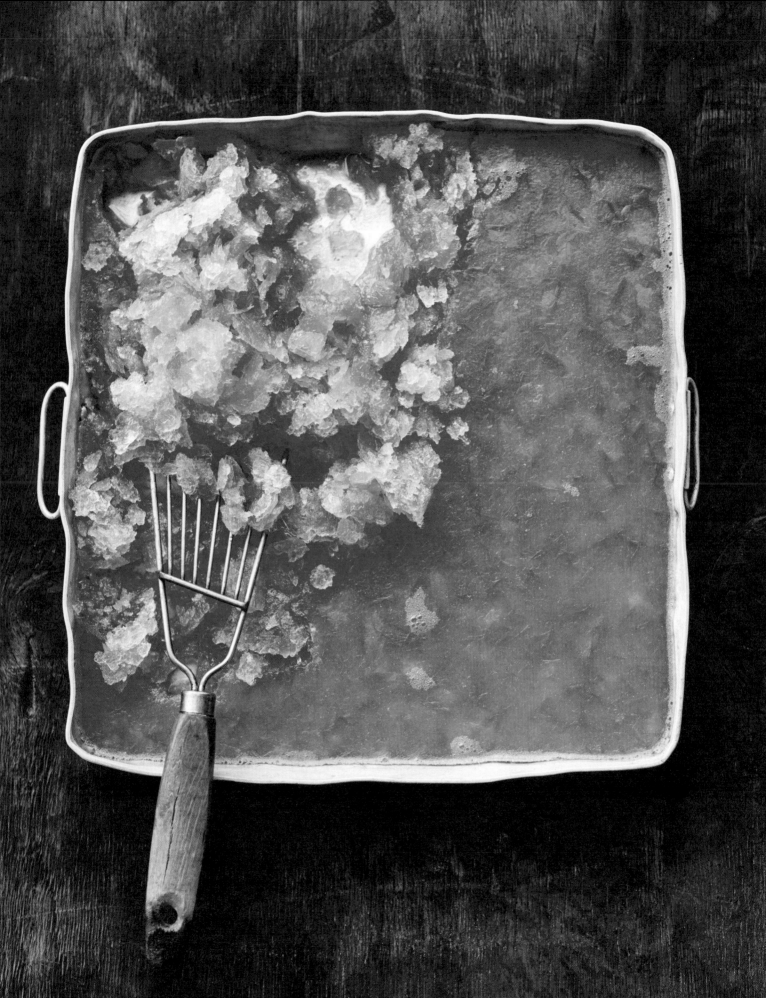

apple CRUMBLES

4 red apples, cored
1 vanilla bean, quartered
crumble filling
⅔ cup (60g/2 oz) rolled oats
¼ cup (30g/1 oz) almond meal (ground almonds)
½ cup (125ml/4¼ fl oz) pure maple syrup
1 teaspoon ground cinnamon
cinnamon and vanilla yoghurt
¾ cup (210g/7½ oz) plain Greek-style (thick) yoghurt
2 teaspoons vanilla bean paste
½ teaspoon ground cinnamon
1 tablespoon pure maple syrup

Preheat oven to 180°C (350°F).

To make the crumble filling, place the oats, almond meal, maple and cinnamon into a bowl and mix to combine.

Place the apples onto a baking tray lined with non-stick baking paper. Use a small sharp knife to score a line around the centre of each apple to stop the apple bursting while baking. Fill the centres of the apples with the crumble mixture. Place remaining mixture under each apple, creating little nests.

Push a piece of the vanilla bean into the centre of the crumble mixture and bake for 20–25 minutes or until the crumble is crisp and the apples are just soft.

While the apples are cooking, make the cinnamon and vanilla yoghurt. In a serving bowl, combine the yoghurt, vanilla, cinnamon and maple.

To serve, place the apple into serving bowls and serve with cinnamon and vanilla yoghurt. **SERVES 4**

I love the look of this inside-out *apple crumble with its vanilla bean stem.* BE GENEROUS when removing the core, so you can pack even more of that crispy CINNAMON filling into the apple.

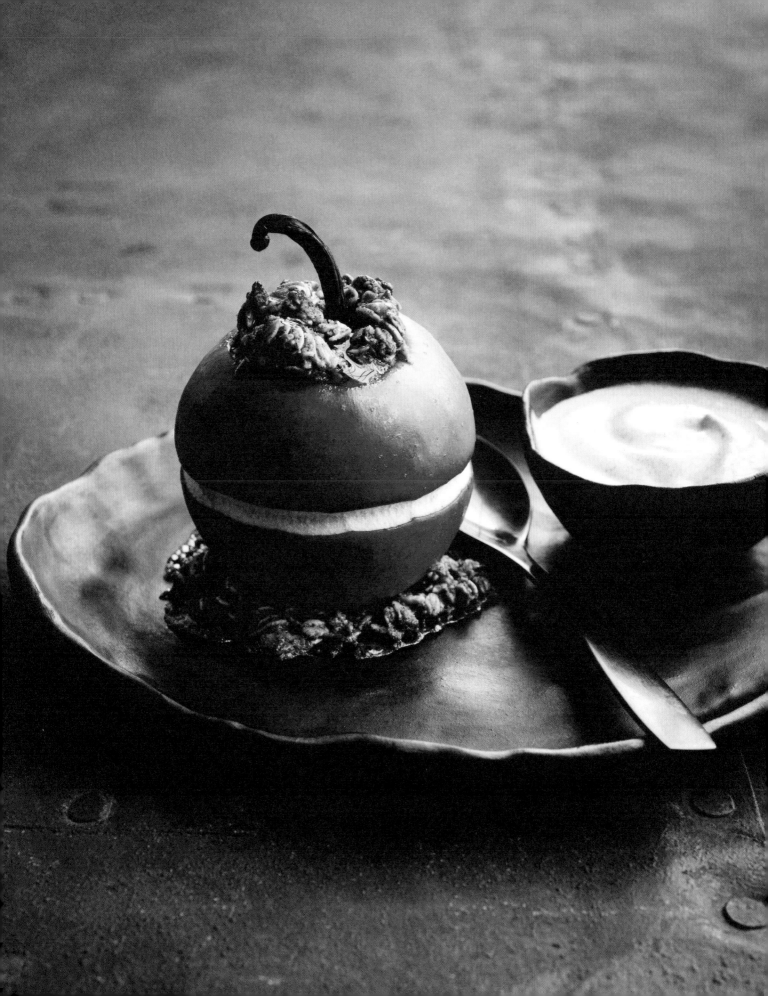

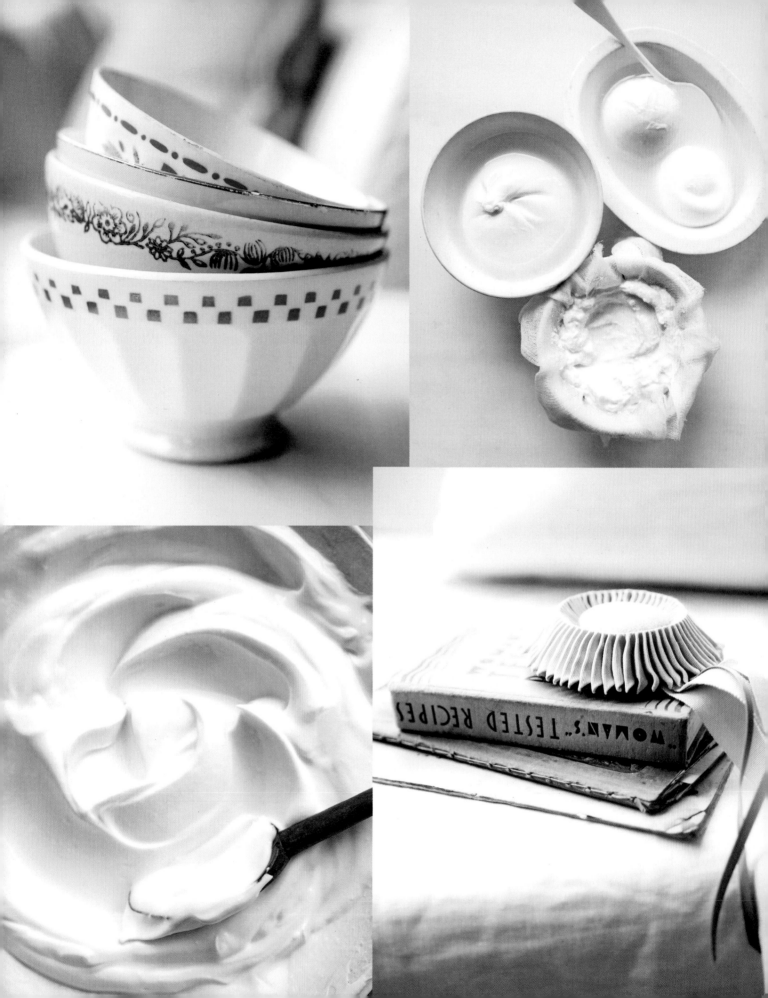

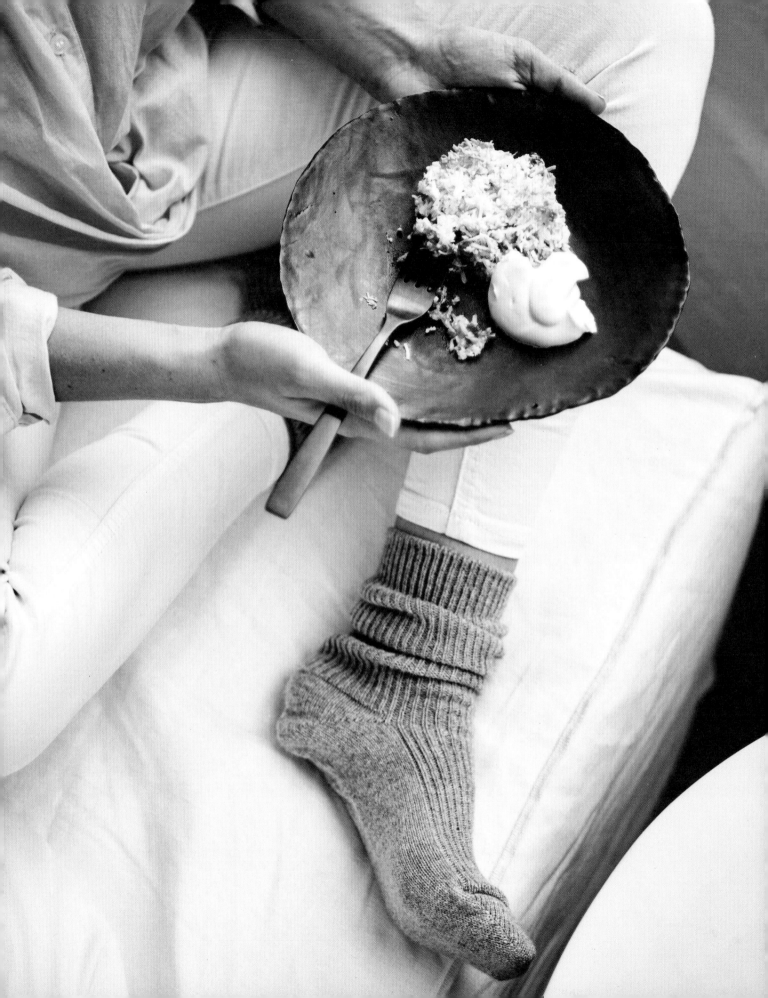

chewy CHOCOLATE
almond *bars*

1 cup (250g/8¾ oz) almond butter
½ cup (125ml/4¼ fl oz) pure maple syrup
½ cup (60g/2 oz) coconut flour
⅓ cup (45g/1½ oz) rolled oats
2 teaspoons vanilla extract
choc-almond topping
180g (6¼ oz) dark (70% cocoa) chocolate, chopped
½ cup (125g/4½ oz) almond butter

Line a 20cm (8 inch) square cake tin with non-stick baking paper,
allowing paper to overhang on all sides.

 Place the almond butter, maple, flour, oats and vanilla in a bowl
and mix to combine. Using the back of a spoon, press mixture into the
prepared tin.

 To make the choc-almond topping, place the chocolate in a heatproof
bowl over a saucepan of simmering water and stir until melted and
smooth. Add the almond butter and stir until combined. Pour the
chocolate over the base and spread evenly. Refrigerate for 1 hour or
until firm. Cut into bars. Store in an airtight container in the fridge.
MAKES 18 BARS

There's nothing like having *a supply of better-for-you
snack bars* on hand for when the MOOD strikes.
This amazingly simple, super-delicious *raw slice
never fails to satisfy* those SWEET CRAVINGS.

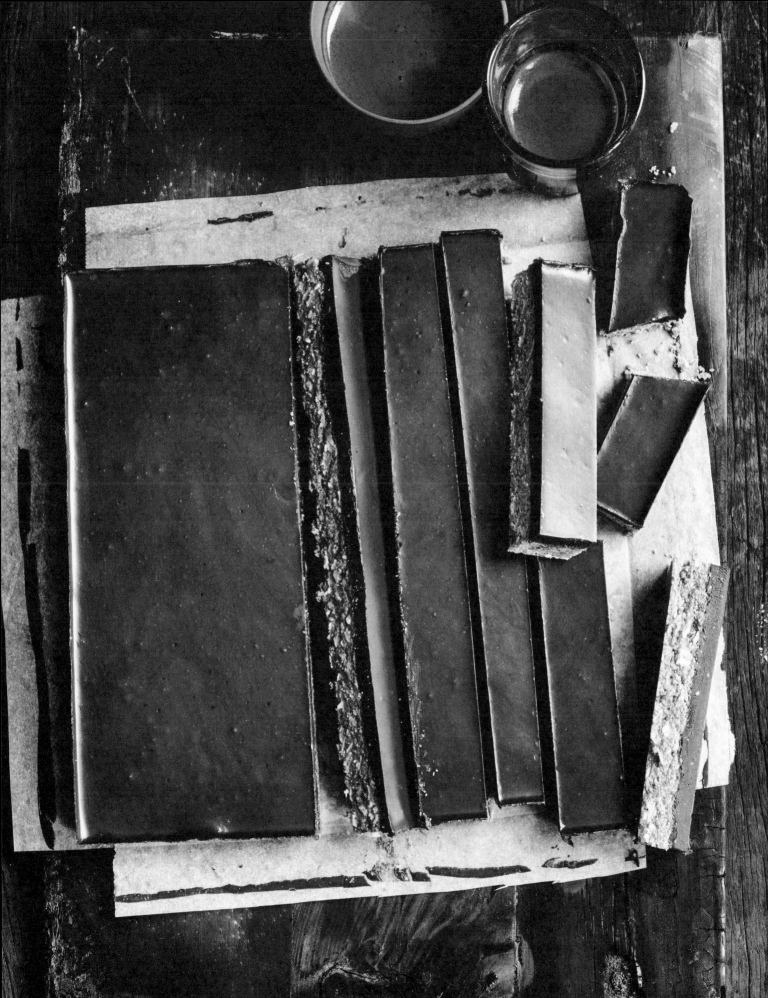

chocolate FUDGE *cake*

¾ cup (180ml/6 fl oz) light-flavoured extra virgin olive oil
½ cup (125ml/4¼ fl oz) milk or nut milk
½ cup (125ml/4¼ fl oz) pure maple syrup
6 eggs
½ cup (110g/4 oz) raw caster (superfine) sugar
2 teaspoons vanilla extract
3 teaspoons baking powder
¾ cup (75g/2½ oz) cocoa powder, sifted
3½ cups (420g/14¾ oz) almond meal (ground almonds)
chocolate frosting
¾ cup (180g/6¼ oz) smooth cashew butter
½ cup (125ml/4¼ fl oz) pure maple syrup
⅓ cup (35g/1¼ oz) cocoa powder, sifted
2 tablespoons milk or nut milk

Preheat oven to 160°C (325°F). Line 2 x 20cm (8 inch) round cake tins with non-stick baking paper.

In a large bowl add oil, milk, maple, eggs, sugar and vanilla into a bowl and whisk to combine.

Sift the baking powder and cocoa over the milk mixture. Add the almond meal and mix to combine. Pour mixture into prepared tins, smoothing the surface. Bake for 30–35 minutes until cooked when tested with a skewer. Cool in tins for 10 minutes then turn out onto wire racks to cool.

To make the chocolate frosting, mix together the cashew butter and maple. Sift over the cocoa powder and stir to combine. Add enough milk to make a spreadable consistency. Using a handheld mixer, beat until smooth.

Spread top of base with half the chocolate frosting. Layer with other cake. Top with remaining frosting. **SERVES 10-12**

It looks and *tastes super-naughty*, but it's actually full of SUPER-NICE (and good-for-you) stuff. This rich, velvety cake topped with *the simplest fudgy icing* will become your go-to CHOCOLATE cake recipe.

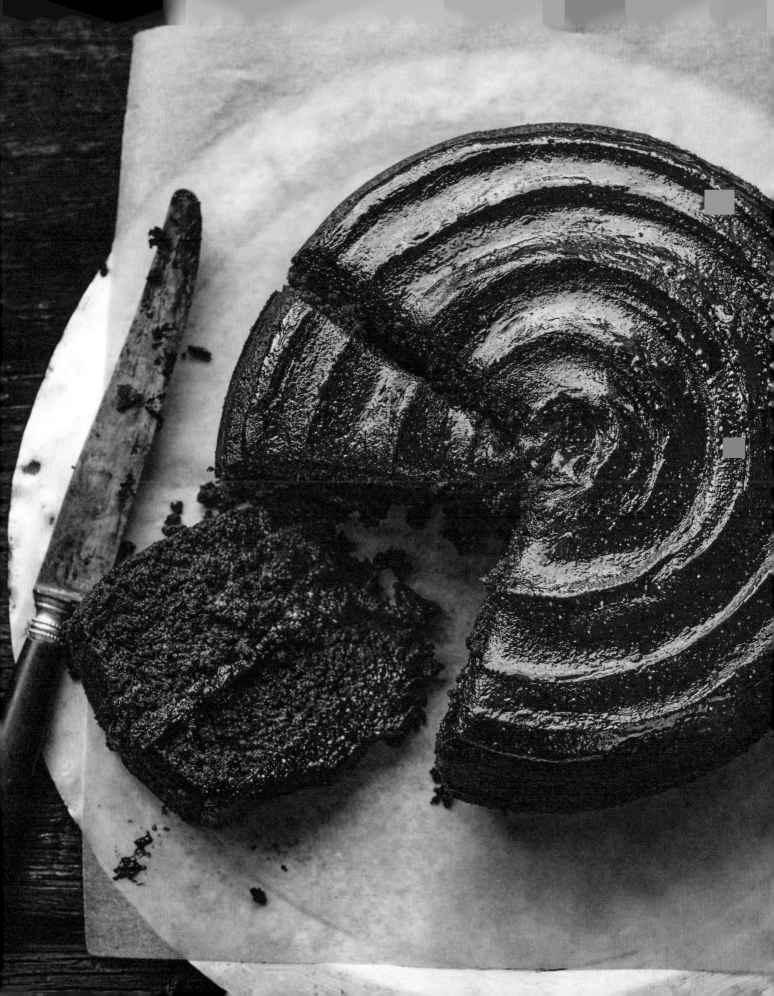

baked CHOCOLATE
tofu *cheesecake*

blueberries, halved, to serve
whipped coconut cream, to serve (optional)
base
⅔ cup (50g/1¾ oz) desiccated coconut
⅔ cup (160g/5½ oz) cashew butter
¼ cup (60ml/2 fl oz) pure maple syrup
filling
500g (1 lb) silken tofu, at room temperature
⅔ cup (160g/5½ oz) firmly packed brown sugar
200g (7 oz) dark (70% cocoa) chocolate, melted and cooled slightly
2 tablespoons cocoa powder
1½ tablespoons cornflour (cornstarch)

Preheat oven to 160°C (325°F). Line a 22cm (8½ inch) round
springform cake tin with non-stick baking paper.

  To make the base, combine the coconut, cashew butter and maple.
Press into the prepared tin and bake for 10 minutes or until lightly
golden brown.

  To make the filling, place the tofu, brown sugar, chocolate, cocoa and
cornflour into the bowl of a food processor and process until smooth.
Pour over the base and bake for 30 minutes or until just set.

  Set aside for 30 minutes, then chill for 2 hours or until cold. Serve
in wedges with blueberries and whipped coconut cream. **SERVES 12**

Don't let the tofu scare you. This cheesecake has a
chocolatey RICH MOUSSE-like texture that is
absolutely amazing. *The perfect recipe to have up
your sleeve* for any vegan or DAIRY-FREE friend.

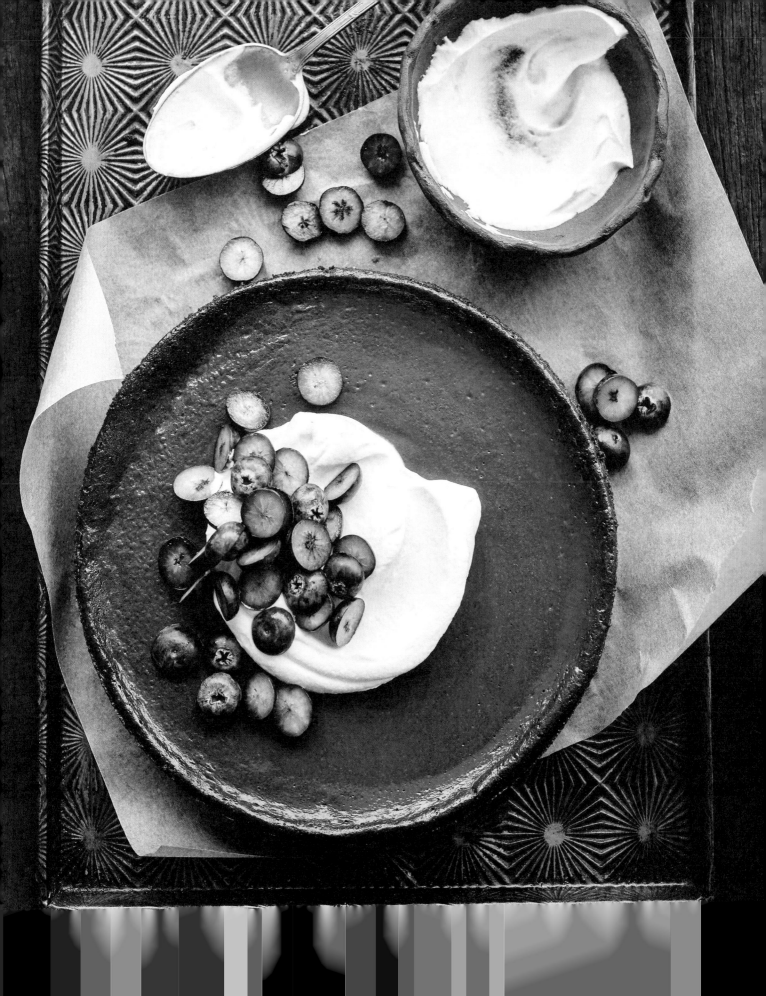

oat AND COCONUT
chocolate *cookie sandwiches*

½ cup (45g/1½ oz) rolled oats
½ cup (40g/1½ oz) desiccated coconut
¾ cup (185g/6½ oz) almond butter
¼ cup (30g/1 oz) almond meal (ground almonds)
½ cup (75g/2¾ oz) coconut sugar
¼ cup (60ml/2 fl oz) pure maple syrup
1 teaspoon vanilla extract
chocolate ganache filling
100g (3½ oz) dark (70% cocoa) chocolate, chopped
¼ cup (60g/2 oz) almond butter

Preheat oven to 160°C (325°F).

Combine oats, coconut, almond butter, almond meal, coconut sugar, maple and vanilla in a bowl and mix well to combine. Roll heaped teaspoons of mixture into balls and place, about 3cm (1 inch) apart, on a tray lined with non-stick baking paper. Flatten slightly.

Bake for 10–12 minutes or until golden brown. Allow to cool on tray.

While biscuits are cooking, make the chocolate ganache filling. Melt the chocolate in a bowl over a saucepan of simmering water. Once melted, stir through the almond butter. Chill for 10 minutes or until it becomes a spreadable consistency.

Sandwich the cooled biscuits together with the ganache and store in an airtight container in the fridge. **MAKES 14 COOKIE SANDWICHES**

These biscuits remind me of a FAVOURITE from my childhood... only way better. *Caramelly, crispy oat cookies* sandwiched with a SMOOTH chocolate filling. *It's hard to stop at just one.*

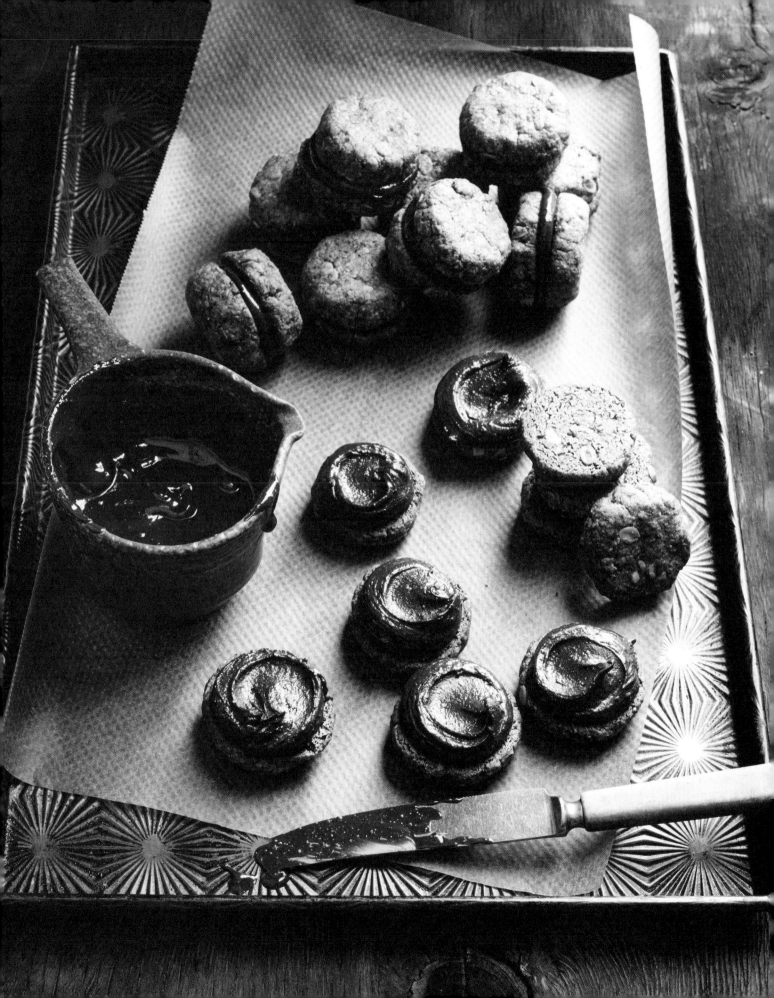

caramelised BANANA
upside down *cake*

2 bananas
⅓ cup (80ml/2¾ fl oz) pure maple syrup, plus extra to serve
cake
1 cup (260g/9 oz) smooth mashed banana (about 3 bananas)
¼ cup (60ml/2 fl oz) milk or nut milk
½ cup (125ml/4¼ fl oz) pure maple syrup
⅔ cup (160ml/5½ fl oz) light-flavoured extra virgin olive oil
3 eggs, lightly whisked
1 teaspoon vanilla extract
2 teaspoons ground cinnamon
1 cup (140g/5 oz) wholemeal (whole-wheat) spelt flour
3 teaspoons baking powder
1 cup (120g/4¼ oz) almond meal (ground almonds)

Preheat oven to 160°C (325°F). Lightly grease a 20cm (8 inch) round cake tin[+] and line with non-stick baking paper.

Peel the bananas and cut into thick slices lengthwise. Pour the maple into the base of the prepared tin and top with the banana slices.

To make the cake, place the mashed banana, milk, maple, oil, egg, vanilla and cinnamon in a large bowl and whisk to combine. Sift over the flour and the baking powder, adding back in the sifted husk. Then add the almond meal and mix to combine. Pour batter over the sliced bananas in the prepared tin.

Bake for 55 minutes or until just cooked when tested with a skewer. Allow cake to cool in tin for 15 minutes. Turn out onto a serving plate and drizzle with extra maple. Serve warm. **SERVES 10-12**

+ *Use a standard round cake tin for this recipe, not a springform cake tin.*

The caramelised MAPLE banana takes the *classic banana cake* to a whole new level of wow with its GOLDEN GLAZE and *syrupy goodness.*

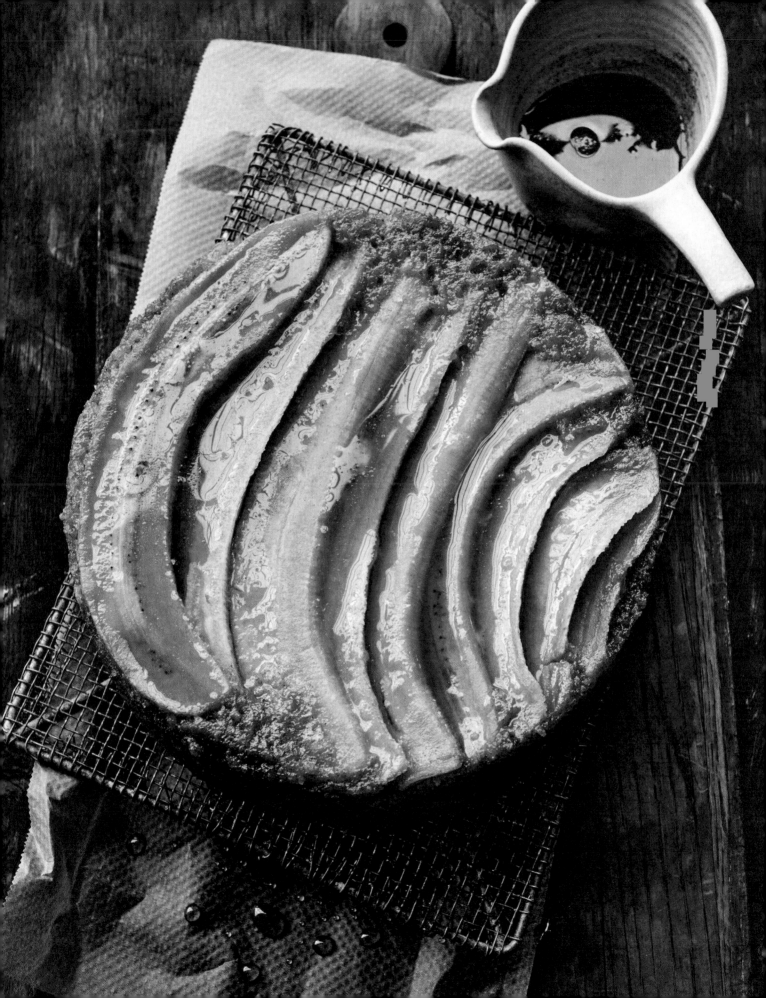

almond CRISP
with *maple pears*

1 cup (120g/4¼ oz) almond meal (ground almonds)
1 cup (95g/3½ oz) flaked almonds
2 egg whites
¼ cup (55g/2 oz) raw caster (superfine) sugar
1 beurre bosc (firm brown) pear
2 tablespoons pure maple syrup
vanilla bean ice-cream or yoghurt, to serve

Preheat oven to 180°C (350°C).

In a medium bowl, place the almond meal, flaked almonds, egg whites and sugar and mix to combine. Divide mixture into 4 and press into 10cm (4 inch) rounds on a baking tray lined with non-stick baking paper. Bake for 10 minutes.

Cut the pear in half vertically and use a teaspoon to remove the core. Cut each half into half again so you have 4 pear quarters. Make 5 slices down the length of each quarter, keeping the top 1cm (½ inch) near the stem intact.

Gently fan out the pear quarters and place 1 on each tart base. Brush pear quarters with maple and bake for 15 minutes or until golden and crispy around the edges.

Brush pears with remaining maple and serve with a scoop of vanilla bean ice-cream. **SERVES 4**

I love that something so simple to make can look and taste SO GOOD. *Sticky wafer-like pear* atop crisp almond biscuits make a PERFECT MATCH.

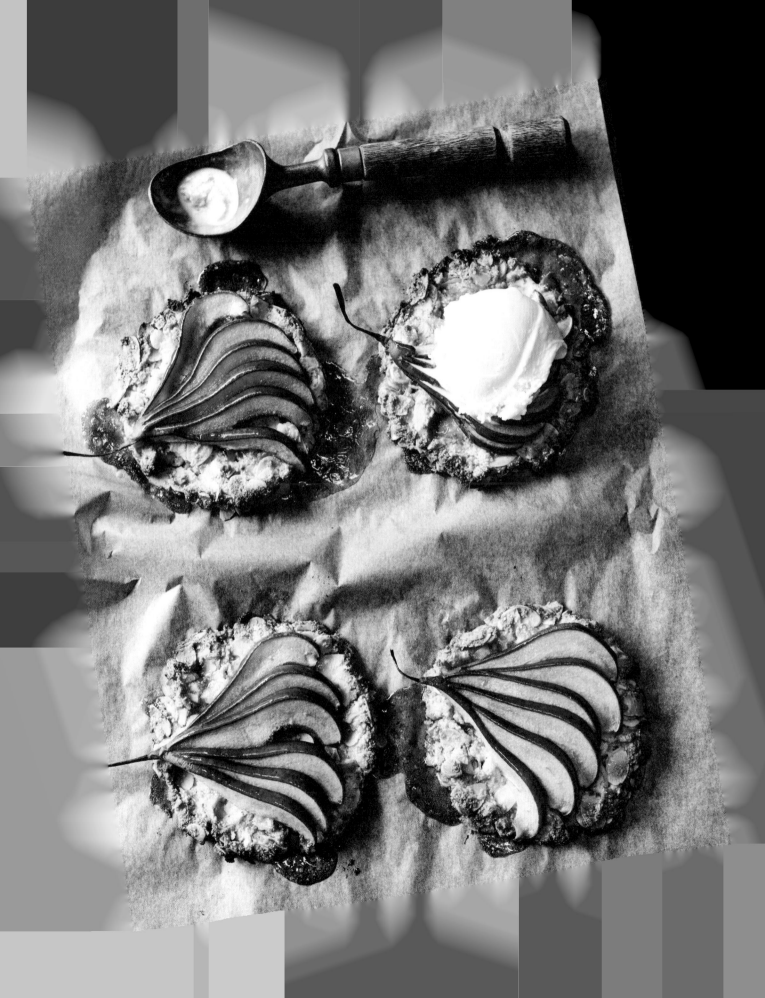

coconut CARAMEL
cashew *bliss balls*

1 cup (250g/8¾ oz) smooth cashew butter
1½ cups (120g/4 oz) desiccated coconut, plus extra for rolling
⅓ cup (80ml/2¾ oz) pure maple syrup
1 teaspoon vanilla extract

Place the cashew butter, coconut, maple and vanilla into a bowl and
mix well to combine. Roll tablespoonfuls into balls and roll in extra
coconut to coat. Store in an airtight container in the refrigerator.
MAKES 20

I wanted to make a SUPER-DELICIOUS bliss ball
recipe that was *lower in sugar* and so wonderfully
SIMPLE that you didn't need a food processor.
Mission accomplished!

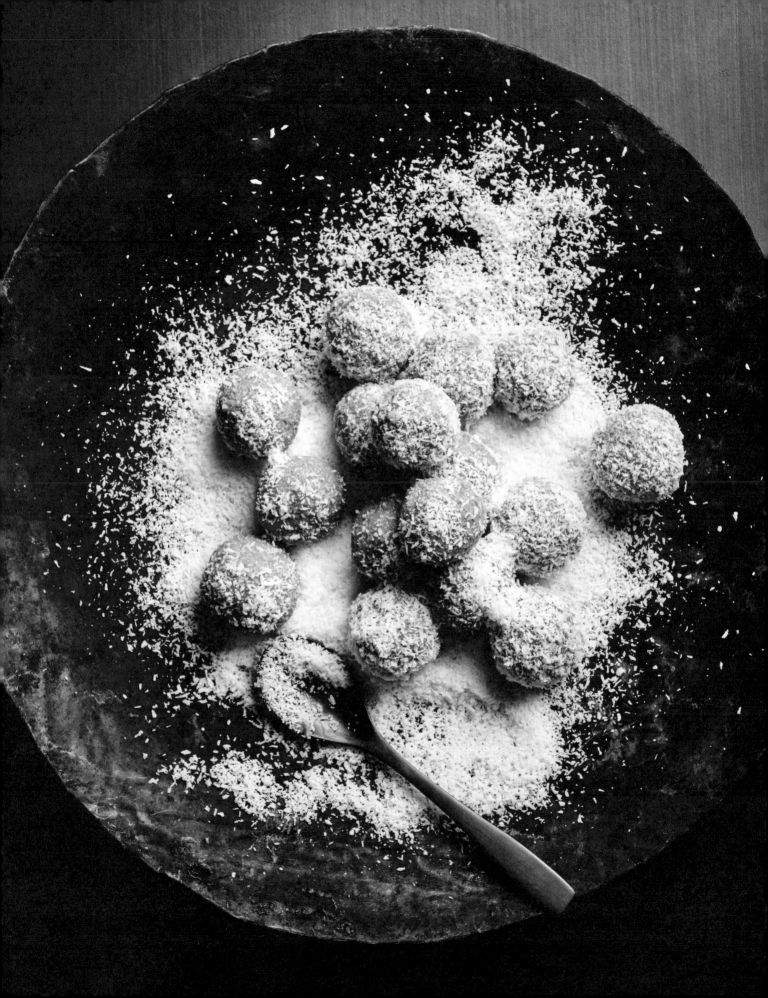

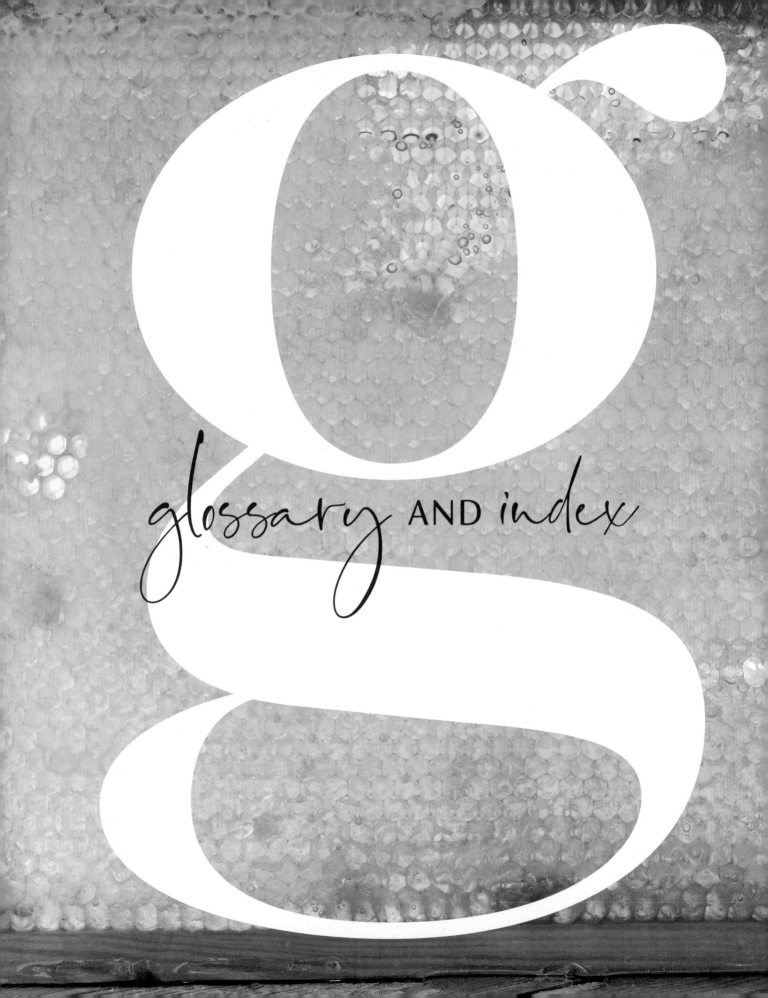

glossary AND index

In the glossary, you'll find basic information on PANTRY STAPLES, plus notes on any of the *unusual ingredients* called for in this book. There are also some really *useful pages* of global measures, temperatures, weights and common conversions. Find all recipes listed alphabetically by name in the index, as well as grouped by their main ingredients.

agave syrup

Agave syrup is the nectar of the agave succulent and has a mild, neutral sweetness. It's often used in place of sugar, maple syrup or honey. It's available from the health food aisle of supermarkets as light or dark agave. Light agave syrup has a milder flavour.

almond butter

This paste is made from ground almonds and is available at most supermarkets and health food stores. It's a popular alternative to peanut butter for those with peanut allergies (always check the label). Sometimes sold as 'spreads', the nut butters called for in this book are all-natural with no additives.

almond meal (ground almonds)

Almond meal is available from most supermarkets. Take care not to confuse it with almond flour, which has a much finer texture. Make your own almond meal by processing whole almonds to a meal in a food processor – 125g (4½ oz) almonds should give 1 cup of almond meal.

baking powder

A raising agent used in baking, consisting of bicarbonate of soda and/or cream of tartar. Most are gluten free (check the label). Baking powder that's kept beyond its use-by date can lose effectiveness.

bicarbonate of (baking) soda

Also known as baking soda, bicarbonate of soda (sodium bicarbonate) is an alkaline powder used to help leaven baked goods and neutralise acids.

blanching

Blanching is a cooking method used to slightly soften the texture, heighten the colour and enhance the flavour of vegetables. Plunge the ingredient briefly into boiling unsalted water, remove and refresh under cold water. Drain well.

bok choy

A mild-flavoured green vegetable, with fresh crunchy white stems and broad floppy green leaves. It's also known as Chinese chard, Chinese white cabbage or pak choy. It's best trimmed, gently steamed, pan-fried or blanched, then teamed with Asian-style rice and noodle dishes or stir-fries.

broccolini (sprouting broccoli)

Also known as tenderstem broccoli, broccolini is a cross between gai lan (Chinese broccoli) and broccoli. This popular green vegetable has long, thin stems and small florets with a slightly sweet flavour. Sold in bunches, it can be substituted with regular heads of broccoli that have been sliced into slim florets.

butter

Unless it says otherwise in a recipe, butter should be at room temperature for cooking. It should not be half-melted or too soft to handle. We mostly prefer unsalted butter, but use salted if you wish.

cabbage

chinese

Also known as wombok or Napa cabbage, Chinese cabbage is elongated in shape with ribbed green-yellow leaves. It's regularly used in noodle salads and to make kimchi. Find it at Asian grocers and greengrocers.

green

Pale green or white with tightly bound, waxy leaves, these common cabbages are sold whole or halved in supermarkets and are perfect for use in slaws. Choose heads that are firm and unblemished with crisp leaves that are tightly packed.

capers

These small green flower buds of the caper bush are packed either in brine or salt. Capers lend their salty-sour intensity to sauces, seafood and pastas. Before using, rinse thoroughly, drain and pat dry.

cashew butter

This paste is made from ground cashews and is available at most supermarkets and health food stores. Often sold as 'spreads', the nut butters called for in this book are all-natural with no additives.

cavolo nero (Tuscan kale)

Translated to mean 'black cabbage', this dark leafy vegetable is similar to silverbeet, and is super nutritious.

cheese

bocconcini

Bite-sized balls of the white fresh mild Italian cheese, mozzarella. Sold in tubs in a lightly salted brine, bocconcini spoils easily so is best consumed within 2–3 days.

buffalo mozzarella

This much-loved variety of fresh Italian mozzarella is made from water buffalo's milk and/or cow's milk. Creamy and salty, it's sold in rounds, or balls, at grocers and delicatessens and is often torn into pieces and scattered over caprese salads or pizza.

burrata
An Italian stretched-curd cheese made from mozzarella, burrata has a creamy, milky centre. It's best served simply, with something like a tomato or fig salad. It's available from delicatessens, specialty cheese stores and Italian grocery stores.

goat's cheese
Goat's milk has a tart flavour, so the cheese made from it, also called chèvre, has a sharp, slightly acidic taste. Immature goat's cheese is mild and creamy and is often labelled goat's curd, which is spreadable. Mature goat's cheese is available in both hard and soft varieties.

haloumi
A firm white Cypriot cheese made from sheep's milk, haloumi has a stringy texture and is usually sold in brine. Slice and pan-fry until golden and heated through for a salty addition to vegies or salads. Buy haloumi at major greengrocers and supermarkets.

marinated feta
Creamy, mild-tasting Greek-style feta has been marinated in oil, often with a mix of herbs, garlic and peppercorns, to make this cheese.

parmesan
Italy's favourite hard, granular cheese is made from cow's milk.

Parmigiano Reggiano is the best variety, made under strict guidelines in the Emilia-Romagna region and aged for an average of two years. Grana Padano mainly comes from Lombardy and is aged for around 15 months.

ricotta
A creamy, finely grained white cheese. Ricotta means 'recooked' in Italian, a reference to the way the cheese is produced by heating the whey leftover from making other cheese varieties. It's fresh, creamy and low in fat and there is also a reduced-fat version, which is lighter again. Choose fresh ricotta from your delicatessen or supermarket deli. Steer away from pre-packaged tubs that are labelled smooth.

chia seeds
These ancient seeds come from a flowering plant and are full of protein, omega-3 fatty acids, minerals and fibre. Use the black or white seeds interchangeably. Find them in supermarkets – they're great for smoothies, salads and baking.

chickpeas (garbanzo beans)
A legume native to western Asia and across the Mediterranean, chickpeas are used in soups, stews and are the base ingredient in hummus. Dried chickpeas need soaking before use; buy them canned to skip this step.

chillies
There are more than 200 different types of chillies, or chilli peppers, in the world. Long red or green chillies are generally milder, fruitier

and sweeter, while small chillies are much hotter. Remove the membranes and seeds for a milder result.

chinese cooking wine (Shaoxing)
Similar to dry sherry, Shaoxing, or Chinese cooking wine, is a blend of glutinous rice, millet, a special yeast and the local spring waters of Shaoxing in northern China, where it is traditionally made. Used in myriad sauces and dressings, it's available from the Asian section of supermarkets and at Asian grocery stores.

coconut
cream
The cream that rises to the top after the first pressing of coconut milk, coconut cream is higher both in energy and fat than regular coconut milk. It's a common ingredient in curries and Asian sweets. You can buy it in cans or cartons from most supermarkets.

desiccated
Desiccated coconut is coconut meat that has been shredded and dried to remove its moisture. It's unsweetened and very powdery. Great for baking as well as savoury Asian sauces and sambals.

flakes
Coconut flakes have a large shape and chewier texture than the desiccated variety, and are often used for decorating and in cereals and baking. You can buy coconut flakes ready-toasted, with lovely golden edges, from supermarkets.

coconut milk
A milky, sweet liquid made by soaking grated fresh coconut flesh or desiccated coconut in warm water and squeezing it through muslin or cheesecloth. Available in cartons or cans from supermarkets, coconut milk shouldn't be confused with coconut water, which is a clear liquid found inside young coconuts. Recipes in this book have been made using coconut milk from cartons, as it tends to be superior in quality.

shredded
In slightly larger pieces than desiccated, shredded coconut is great for adding a bit more texture to slices and cakes, or for making condiments to serve with curries.

sugar
See *sugar (coconut)*, page 214.

yoghurt
Coconut yoghurt has become far more readily available in recent years, thanks to its dairy-free status. It's made from coconut milk and probiotic cultures. Find it in the chilled yoghurt section of most supermarkets and in specialty grocers and health food stores.

coriander (cilantro)
This pungent green herb is common in Asian and Mexican cooking. The finely chopped roots are sometimes incorporated into curry pastes. The dried seeds can't be substituted for fresh coriander.

dark chocolate
The dark chocolate called for in this book is 65–70% cocoa solids.

Chocolate that has 70% cocoa solids is usually labelled as such, and has a more bitter, intense flavour and no powdery texture. It's sold in blocks and is ideal for use in baking. Find it in the baking aisle of supermarkets.

dukkah
A Middle-Eastern nut and spice blend available from some supermarkets, from spice shops and specialty grocery stores. Great for sprinkling on meats and salads or using in a spice crust.

edamame
Find these tasty, tender soy beans ready-podded in the freezer section of major greengrocers, Asian grocers and some supermarkets.

eggs
The standard egg size used in this book is 60g (2 oz). It's important to use the right sized eggs, for baking recipes especially, as it can affect the outcome. Room temperature eggs are best for baking.

fish sauce
This amber-coloured liquid drained from salted, fermented fish is used to add flavour to Thai and Vietnamese dishes, such as curries, plus dressings and dipping sauces.

flour
buckwheat
Despite its name, buckwheat flour isn't from a grain but is milled from the seed of a plant related to rhubarb and sorrel. Often used in pancakes and noodles for its rich, nutty flavour and wholesome benefits, it's also gluten free.

cornflour (cornstarch)
When made from ground corn or maize, cornflour is gluten free. Recipes often require it to be blended with water or stock for a thickening agent. Not to be confused with cornflour in the United States, which is finely ground corn meal.

plain (all-purpose)
Ground from the endosperm of wheat, plain white flour contains no raising agent.

rice
Rice flour is a fine flour made from ground rice. Available in white and brown varieties, it's often used as a thickening agent in baking, in cookies and shortbreads, and to coat foods when cooking Asian dishes. It's gluten free and available in supermarkets and health food stores.

self-raising (self-rising)
Ground from the endosperm of wheat, self-raising flour contains raising agents including sodium carbonates and calcium phosphates.

spelt
Milled from the ancient cereal grain, spelt flour boasts more nutrients and is better tolerated by some than regular flour.

wholemeal (whole-wheat)
Ground from the whole grain of wheat and thus keeping more of its nutrients and fibre, this flour is available in plain (all-purpose) and self-raising (self-rising) varieties from most supermarkets and health food stores.

freekeh

Freekeh is the immature or 'green' wheat grain that's been roasted. The recipes in this book call for whole-grain freekeh as opposed to cracked freekeh. The grains can be used in salads and tabouli or eat it as you would rice or pasta. Find it in supermarkets and health food stores. 1 cup cooked freekeh weighs 160g (5½ oz). Directions for cooking freekeh are as follows.

1 cup (220g/7¾ oz) freekeh
3 cups (750ml/25 fl oz) water

Place the freekeh and water in a medium saucepan over high heat. Bring to the boil, immediately cover with a tight-fitting lid and reduce the heat to low. Cook for 30–35 minutes or until tender. Drain any remaining water.
MAKES 3 CUPS (480G/1 LB)

gai lan (chinese broccoli)

Also known as Chinese broccoli or Chinese kale, gai lan is a leafy vegetable with dark green leaves, tiny white or yellow flowers and stout stems. It can be steamed or blanched and served with oyster sauce as a simple side or added to soups, stir-fries and braises towards the end of the cooking time. Gai lan is sold in bunches at greengrocers and supermarkets.

green onions (scallions)

Both the white and green part of these long mild onions are used in salads, as a garnish and in Asian cooking. Sold in bunches, they give a fresh bite to dishes.

harissa

A North-African condiment, harissa is a hot red paste made from chilli, garlic and spices including coriander, caraway and cumin. It can also contain tomato. Available in jars and tubes from supermarkets and specialty food stores, harissa enlivens tagines and couscous dishes. Add it to dressings and sauces for an instant flavour kick.

hoisin sauce

This thick, sweet and salty sauce is used extensively in Chinese cuisine. It is a dark soy-based sauce that can be used as a glaze, in sauces and as a dipping sauce. Find it in the Asian aisle in the supermarket.

horseradish

A pungent root vegetable that releases mustard oil when cut or grated, horseradish is available fresh from greengrocers. You can substitute it with pre-grated or creamed varieties sold in jars.

kaffir lime leaves

Fragrant leaves from the kaffir lime tree have a distinctive double-leaf structure. Commonly crushed or shredded and used in Thai dishes, the leaves are available, fresh or dried, from most greengrocers and at Asian food stores. Fresh leaves are more flavourful and freeze well.

kecap manis

Also know as sweet soy sauce, kecap manis or ketjap manis is a type of soy sauce that originated in Indonesia. It is thicker and sweeter than soy sauce. Find it in the Asian food section of most supermarkets.

labne

A soft, fresh cheese made from strained yoghurt. Find this creamy Middle-Eastern cheese in tubs in the chilled section of greengrocers, gourmet food stores and some supermarkets.

lemongrass

Lemongrass is a tall lemon-scented grass used in Asian cooking, mainly in Thai dishes. Peel away the outer leaves and chop the tender white root-end finely, or add in large pieces during cooking and remove before serving. If adding in larger pieces, bruise them with the back of a kitchen knife.

maple syrup

A sweetener made from the sap of the maple tree, be sure to use pure maple syrup. Imitation, or pancake, syrup is made from corn syrup flavoured with maple and does not have the same intensity of flavour.

mirin (japanese rice wine)

Mirin is a pale yellow, sweet and tangy Japanese cooking wine made from glutinous rice and alcohol.

miso paste

Miso is a traditional Japanese ingredient produced by fermenting rice, barley or soy beans to a paste. It's used for sauces and spreads, pickling vegetables, and is often mixed with dashi stock to serve as miso soup. Sometimes labelled simply 'miso', white, yellow and red varieties are available, their flavour increasing in intensity with their colour. The recipes in this book call for white miso (shiro) for its delicate flavour and colour. Find miso paste in supermarkets and Asian grocers.

noodles

Keep a supply of dried noodles in the pantry for last-minute meals. Most fresh noodles will keep in the fridge for up to a week. Available from supermarkets and Asian food stores.

cellophane (bean thread)

Also called mung bean vermicelli or glass noodles, these noodles are very thin and almost transparent. Soak them in boiling water and drain well to prepare for use.

dried rice

Fine, dried (stick) noodles common in southeast Asian cooking. Depending on their thickness, rice noodles need only be boiled briefly, or soaked in hot water until soft.

rice vermicelli

Very thin dried rice noodles sometimes called rice sticks. They are usually used in soups such as laksa and in salads.

soba

Japanese noodles made from buckwheat and wheat flour, soba are greyish brown in colour and served in cold salads or in hot soups.

udon

This thick Japanese wheat noodle is commonly used in soups.

nori

Nori sheets are paper-thin layers of dried seaweed, commonly used for making sushi rolls. High in protein and minerals, nori can also be chopped, added to soups or used as a garnish. Buy nori, ready-toasted if necessary, at most supermarkets, at greengrocers and Asian grocers.

nutritional yeast

This is inactive yeast that is grown specifically to be used in food. It is a complete protein, so it's a great addition to a vegan diet. Nutritional yeast is called as such because it contains essential vitamins and minerals – it's high in B vitamins. It adds a savoury, umami flavour to dishes. Find it in the health food section of most supermarkets.

oil

extra virgin olive

Graded according to its flavour, aroma and acidity. Extra virgin is the highest-quality olive oil; it contains no more than 1% acid. Virgin is the next best; it contains 1.5% or less acid. Bottles labelled simply 'olive oil' contain a blend of refined and unrefined virgin olive oil. 'Light' olive oil is the least pure in quality and shouldn't be confused with light-flavoured extra virgin olive oil.

light-flavoured extra virgin olive

This is still the highest-quality olive oil and is made from a pure blend of the oil from milder-flavoured olives.

grapeseed

A by-product of winemaking, grapeseed oil is made using the pressed seeds of grapes. It has a suprisingly neutral flavour. Choose grapeseed oil that has been cold-pressed or expeller pressed. Find it in most supermarkets.

sesame

Pressed from sesame seeds, sesame oil is used in Asian cuisine more as a nutty, full-flavoured seasoning than a cooking medium.

vegetable

Oils sourced from plants or seeds, with very mild, unobtrusive flavours. Often called for in baking recipes, such as muffins or loaf cakes, for this reason.

paprika, smoked

Unlike Hungarian paprika, the Spanish style, known as pimentón, is deep and smoky in flavour. It is made from smoked, ground pimento peppers and comes in varying intensities, from sweet and mild (dulce), bittersweet medium hot (agridulce) and hot (picante). The variety called for in this book is smoky-sweet.

pastry

Make your own or use one of the many store-bought varieties, including shortcrust and filo, which are sold frozen in blocks or ready-rolled into pastry sheets. Defrost in the fridge before use.

puff and butter puff

This pastry is quite difficult to make, so many cooks opt to use store-bought puff pastry. It can be bought in blocks from patisseries, or sold in both block and sheet forms in supermarkets. Butter puff pastry is very light and flaky, perfect for both savoury and sweet pies and tarts. Often labelled 'all butter puff', good-quality sheets are usually thicker. If you can only buy thin sheets of butter puff, don't be afraid to stack 2 regular thawed sheets together.

pepitas (pumpkin seeds)

Pumpkin seeds are hulled to reveal these olive green kernels that, once dried, are nutty in flavour and easy to use in smoothies, baking and salads. Find them in supermarkets.

pickled ginger

Also known as gari, this Japanese condiment is made from young ginger that's been pickled in sugar and vinegar. It's commonly served with Japanese food as a palate cleanser, but is becoming popular as a tangy addition to sushi bowls and salads. Buy it in jars from Asian grocers and some supermarkets.

pomegranate molasses

A concentrated syrup made from pomegranate juice, with a sweet, tart flavour, pomegranate molasses is available from Middle Eastern grocery stores and specialty food shops. If you can't find it, try using caramelised balsamic vinegar.

quinoa

Packed with protein, this grain-like seed has a chewy texture, nutty flavour and is fluffy when cooked. Use it as you would couscous or rice. It freezes well, so any excess cooked quinoa can be frozen in individual portions. Red and black varieties, which require a slightly longer cooking time, are also available in most supermarkets. 1 cup cooked white quinoa weighs 160g (5½ oz). Directions for cooking quinoa are as follows.

1 cup (180g/6¼ oz) white quinoa
1¼ cups (310ml/10½ fl oz) water
sea salt flakes

Place the quinoa, water and a pinch of salt in a medium saucepan over high heat. Bring to the boil, cover immediately with a tight-fitting lid and reduce the heat to low. Simmer for 12 minutes or until almost tender. Remove from the heat and allow to steam for 8 minutes or until tender. **MAKES 2¾ CUPS (440G/15½ OZ)**

flakes

Quinoa flakes are simply quinoa seeds that have been steamrolled into flakes. Use them in breakfast cereals or baked goods. Find them in health food stores and the health food aisle of supermarkets.

raw cacao

Available in nibs and powder form, raw cacao comes from tropical cacao beans that have been cold pressed. Rich, dark and pleasantly bitter; find it in health food stores and supermarkets.

rice

aborio

Rice with a short, plump-looking grain that cooks to a soft texture, while retaining a firm interior. It has surface starch that creates a creamy texture in risottos when cooked to al dente. Available at specialty food stores and most supermarkets.

black

This highly nutritious rice is also known as the forbidden rice, because it was once reserved for Chinese royalty and forbidden to anyone else. The black colour of the rice is due to its high levels of the antioxidant anthocyanin. Black rice also contains more protein than any other rice variety and is a good source of iron.

1½ cups black rice
3½ cups (875ml/29½ fl oz) water

Place the rice and water in a medium saucepan over high heat. Bring to the boil. Cover with a tight-fitting lid, reduce heat to low and cook for 35 minutes or until tender. **MAKES 4½ CUPS (875G/1 LB 9 OZ)**

brown

Brown rice is different to white rice in that the bran and germ of the wholegrain are intact. This renders it nutritionally superior and gives it a nutty chewiness. 1 cup cooked brown rice weighs 200g (7 oz). Directions for cooking brown rice are as follows.

1 cup (200g/7 oz) brown rice
1½ cups (375ml/12½ fl oz) water
sea salt flakes

Place the rice, water and a pinch of salt in a medium saucepan over high heat. Bring to the boil, immediately cover with a tight-fitting lid and reduce the heat to low. Simmer for 25 minutes or until almost tender. Remove from the heat and allow to steam for 10 minutes or until tender. **MAKES 2 CUPS (400G/14 OZ)**

sashimi-grade fish

Sashimi-grade means the freshest fish available. They are line-caught and therefore have no bruises. It's best to buy a centre piece from the fillet as it won't have veins, skin or blood lines. To ensure freshness, you should buy your fish from the market the day you're going to eat it. Pop it into the freezer for 20 minutes before thinly slicing.

sage

This Mediterranean herb has a distinct, fragrant flavour and soft, oval-shaped grey-green leaves. It's used often in Italian cooking, crisped in a pan with butter or oil.

sesame seeds

These small seeds have a nutty flavour and can be used in savoury and sweet cooking. White sesame seeds are the most common variety, but black, or unhulled, seeds are popular for coatings in Asian cooking.

shiso leaves

Sometimes called perilla, this herb comes in both green and purple-leafed varieties. It has a slight peppery flavour and is often used to wrap ingredients. The micro variety makes a pretty garnish. Find it at some greengrocers and Asian markets.

silverbeet (swiss chard)

A vegetable with large, crinkly, glossy dark green leaves and prominent white, red or yellow stalks, silverbeet is rich in nutrients. It can be used in salads, soups, pies and steamed as a side. Not to be confused with English spinach which has a smaller and more delicate leaf, silverbeet is best trimmed and washed before use.

sorrel leaves

This leafy green has a signature sour flavour. The red-veined leaves are a pretty and nutritious addition to salads. Find red-veined sorrel leaves at your local greengrocer.

sriracha hot chilli sauce

A hot sauce containing chilli, salt, sugar, vinegar and garlic, sriracha is both the brand name of a popular American blend as well as the generic name for the Southeast-Asian sauce. Use sriracha as a condiment or in marinades. Find it in supermarkets.

sugar

Extracted as crystals from the juice of the sugar cane plant, sugar is a sweetener, flavour enhancer and food preservative.

brown

In Australia, what is known as 'brown sugar' is referred to as 'light brown sugar' in other parts of the world. Light and dark brown sugars are made from refined sugar with natural molasses added. The amount, or percentage, of molasses in relation to the sugar determines its classification as dark or light. The molasses gives the sugar a smooth caramel flavour and also a soft, slightly moist texture. Light and dark types are interchangeable if either is unavailable. An important ingredient in cookies, puddings, dense cakes and brownies, you can find both varieties of brown sugar in supermarkets.

caster (superfine)

The superfine granule of caster sugar gives baked products a light texture and crumb, which is important for many cakes and delicate desserts. Caster sugar is essential for making meringue, as the fine crystals dissolve more easily in the whipped eggwhite.

coconut

With an earthy, butterscotch flavour, coconut sugar, or coconut palm sugar, comes from the flowers of the coconut palm. Coconut sugar gives a lovely depth of flavour. Find it in some supermarkets, specialty food shops, Asian grocers and health food stores.

raw (golden) caster

Light brown in colour and honey-like in flavour, raw sugar is slightly less refined than white sugar, with a larger granule. It lends a more pronounced flavour and colour to baked goods. You can use demerara sugar in its place.

white (granulated)

Regular granulated sugar is used in baking when a light texture is not crucial. The crystals are larger, so you need to beat, add liquids to or heat this sugar if you want to dissolve it.

sumac

These dried berries of a flowering plant are ground to produce an acidic, vibrant crimson powder that's popular in the Middle East. Sumac has a lemony flavour and is great sprinkled on salads, dips or chicken. Find it at specialty spice shops, greengrocers and some supermarkets.

sunflower seeds

These small grey kernels from the black and white seeds of sunflowers are mostly processed for their oil. The kernels are also found in snack mixes and muesli, and can be baked into breads and slices. Buy sunflower seeds in supermarkets.

tahini

A thick paste made from ground sesame seeds, tahini is widely used in Middle-Eastern cooking. It's available in jars and cans from supermarkets and health food stores, in both hulled and unhulled varieties. The recipes in this book call for hulled tahini, for its slightly smoother texture.

tamari

This Japanese sauce is also known as gluten-free soy sauce. Tamari is slightly darker and thicker than soy sauce and has a more balanced flavour. Most tamari sauces are gluten free, however always check the bottle. Find it in the Asian section of the supermarket.

tofu

Not all tofu is created equal. The recipes in this book call for either firm or silken tofu, which can be found in the chilled section of the supermarket. Where possible, choose organic non-GMO tofu. All brands vary in texture and taste, so don't give up until you find one you love. It's a great source of protein and acts like a sponge for flavour.

vanilla

bean paste

This store-bought paste is a convenient way to replace whole vanilla beans and is great in desserts. One teaspoon of paste substitutes for one vanilla bean.

beans

These fragrant cured pods from the vanilla orchid are used whole, often split and the tiny seeds inside scraped into the mixture to infuse flavour into custard and cream-based recipes. They offer a rich and rounded vanilla flavour.

extract

For a pure vanilla taste, use a good-quality vanilla extract, not an essence or imitation flavour.

vincotto

Translating literally as 'cooked wine', vincotto is a syrup made from grapes with a sharp, sweet-sour flavour. Use it as you would balsamic vinegar. Find it in the condiment section of supermarkets and specialty grocers.

vinegar

apple cider

Made from apple must, cider vinegar has a golden amber hue and a sour appley flavour. Use it to make dressings, marinades and chutneys. The recipes in this book call for organic or unfiltered apple cider vinegar.

balsamic

Originally from Modena in Italy, there are many balsamics on the market ranging in quality and flavour. Aged varieties are preferable. A milder white version is also available, which is used where colour is important.

wine

Both red and white wine can be distilled into vinegar. Use in dressings, glazes and preserved condiments such as pickles. Use it to make a classic French vinaigrette.

rice wine

Made from fermenting rice (or rice wine), rice wine vinegar is milder and sweeter than vinegars that are made by oxidising distilled wine or other alcohol made from grapes. Rice wine vinegar is available in white, black, brown and red varieties from supermarkets and Asian food stores.

wasabi paste

We know this Japanese paste for its powdery green colour and its heat. Similar to (and most-likely containing) horseradish, wasabi paste is used as an ingredient and popular condiment for sushi. It's sold, usually in tubes, at Asian grocers and supermarkets.

xanthan gum

A natural, vegan food thickener and stabiliser similar to gelatin, xathan gum is sold as a powder. Use it to thicken ice-creams and in gluten-free baking to help improve elasticity. Available in supermarkets.

yoghurt, natural Greek-style

Recipes in this book call for natural, unsweetened full-fat Greek-style (thick) yoghurt. Buy it from the chilled aisle of the supermarket, checking the label for any unwanted sweeteners or artificial flavours.

global measures

Measures vary from Europe to the US and even from Australia to New Zealand.

metric and imperial

Measuring cups and spoons may vary slightly from one country to another, but the difference is generally not sufficient to affect a recipe. The recipes in this book use Australian measures (with American conversions). All cup and spoon measures are level. An Australian measuring cup holds 250ml (8½ fl oz).

One Australian metric teaspoon holds 5ml (⅛ fl oz), one Australian tablespoon holds 20ml (¾ fl oz) (4 teaspoons). However, in the USA, New Zealand and the UK, 15ml (½ fl oz) (3-teaspoon) tablespoons are used.

If measuring liquid ingredients, remember that 1 American pint contains 475ml (16 fl oz) but 1 imperial pint contains 570ml (19 fl oz).

When measuring dry ingredients, add the ingredient loosely to the cup and level with a knife. Don't tap or shake to compact the ingredient unless the recipe requests 'firmly packed'.

liquids and solids

Measuring cups, spoons and scales are great assets in the kitchen – these equivalents are a guide.

liquids

cup	metric	imperial
⅛ cup	30ml	1 fl oz
¼ cup	60ml	2 fl oz
⅓ cup	80ml	2¾ fl oz
½ cup	125ml	4¼ fl oz
⅔ cup	160ml	5½ fl oz
¾ cup	180ml	6 fl oz
1 cup	250ml	8½ fl oz
2 cups	500ml	17 fl oz
3 cups	750ml	25 fl oz
4 cups	1 litre	34 fl oz

solids

metric	imperial
20g	¾ oz
60g	2 oz
125g	4½ oz
180g	6¼ oz
250g	8¾ oz
450g	1 lb
750g	1 lb 10 oz
1kg	2 lb 3 oz

more equivalents

Here are a few more simplified equivalents for metric and imperial measures, plus ingredient names.

millimetres to inches

metric	imperial
3mm	⅛ inch
6mm	¼ inch
1cm	½ inch
2.5cm	1 inch
5cm	2 inches
18cm	7 inches
20cm	8 inches
23cm	9 inches
25cm	10 inches
30cm	12 inches

ingredient equivalents

almond meal	ground almonds
bicarbonate of soda	baking soda
caster sugar	superfine sugar
celeriac	celery root
chickpeas	garbanzo beans
coriander	cilantro
cornflour	cornstarch
cos lettuce	romaine lettuce
eggplant	aubergine
gai lan	chinese broccoli
green onion	scallion
icing sugar	confectioner's sugar
plain flour	all-purpose flour
rocket	arugula
self-raising flour	self-rising flour
silverbeet	swiss chard
snow pea	mange tout
white sugar	granulated sugar
zucchini	courgette

oven temperatures

Setting the oven to the correct temperature can be crucial when baking sweet things.

celsius to fahrenheit

celsius	fahrenheit
100°C	200°F
120°C	250°F
140°C	275°F
150°C	300°F
160°C	325°F
180°C	350°F
190°C	375°F
200°C	400°F
220°C	425°F

electric to gas

celsius	gas
110°C	¼
130°C	½
140°C	1
150°C	2
170°C	3
180°C	4
190°C	5
200°C	6
220°C	7
230°C	8
240°C	9
250°C	10

butter and eggs

Let 'fresh is best' be your mantra when it comes to selecting eggs and dairy goods.

butter

We generally use unsalted butter as it allows for a little more control over a recipe's flavour. Either way, the impact is minimal. Salted butter has a longer shelf life and is preferred by some people. One American stick of butter is 125g (4½ oz). One Australian block of butter is 250g (8¾ oz).

eggs

Unless otherwise indicated, we use large (60g/2 oz) chicken eggs. To preserve freshness, store eggs in the refrigerator in the carton they are sold in. Use only the freshest eggs in recipes such as mayonnaise or dressings that use raw or barely cooked eggs. Be extra cautious if there is a salmonella problem in your community, particularly in food that is to be served to children, pregnant women or the elderly.

useful weights

Here are a few simple weight conversions for cupfuls of commonly used ingredients.

common ingredients

almond meal (ground almonds)
1 cup | 120g | 4¼ oz
brown sugar
1 cup | 175g | 6 oz
white (granulated) sugar
1 cup | 220g | 7¾ oz
caster (superfine) sugar
1 cup | 220g | 7¾ oz
icing (confectioner's) sugar
1 cup | 160g | 5½ oz
**plain (all-purpose)
or self-raising (self-rising) flour**
1 cup | 150g | 5¼ oz
fresh breadcrumbs
1 cup | 70g | 2½ oz
finely grated parmesan
1 cup | 80g | 2¾ oz
uncooked white rice
1 cup | 200g | 7 oz
cooked white rice
1 cup | 165g | 5¾ oz
uncooked couscous
1 cup | 200g | 7 oz
**cooked shredded chicken,
pork or beef**
1 cup | 160g | 5½ oz
olives
1 cup | 150g | 5¼ oz

thank you

It takes a team of exceptional talent to make a cookbook come together. Never before in my career has a book been created under such unprecedented circumstances. I'm so grateful to the following people for their dedication and can-do approach to everything life throws at them.

Con Poulos – such quiet dedication. From beautiful light falling across these images, to your calming patience and dedication to creating the perfect shot. Every day I spend in the studio with you is an absolute treat.

Hannah Schubert – when I read your credit as senior designer, I feel the need to add recipe note taker, taste tester, production and studio manager and twinkling magic maker. My heartfelt thanks for the many hats you so effortlessly wear, your attention to every perfect detail and for keeping us on track. You are the most fabulous book creator. Big thanks.

Genevieve McKelvey, my trusted creative director – your very fine touch is always very much appreciated.

Dani Bertollo, my editor – so comforting to have such a passionate foodie with a wealth of knowledge and experience on the team.

Peta Dent, Madeleine Jeffreys, Sarah Watson, Sandy Goh, Melissa Burge. I really appreciate all your creative talents (laughs and good times) and precision in the kitchen. You are the ultimate back-up dancers! Take a bow.

At HarperCollinsPublishers, I absolutely need to thank Catherine Milne, Janelle Garside and Belinda Yuille for their ongoing dedication and faith in me.

Thank you to my loyal brand partners: Smeg, Cobram Estate and Cloudy Bay. My gratitude to ceramicist Marjoke De Heer in Amsterdam – your beautiful pieces have made this book shine. Such a generous and kind spirit. MCM House – thank you for my lifestyle furnishings.

To the dh dream team: Karen Hay – all things finance and numbers (a creative girl's dream). Morgan Lee – sponsorship and collaborations manager who can pivot to supermodel in an instant. What a talent!

Last but not least, huge thank yous to all of my boys, big and little, my family and my amazing friends – you give me all the support and love a girl could wish for.

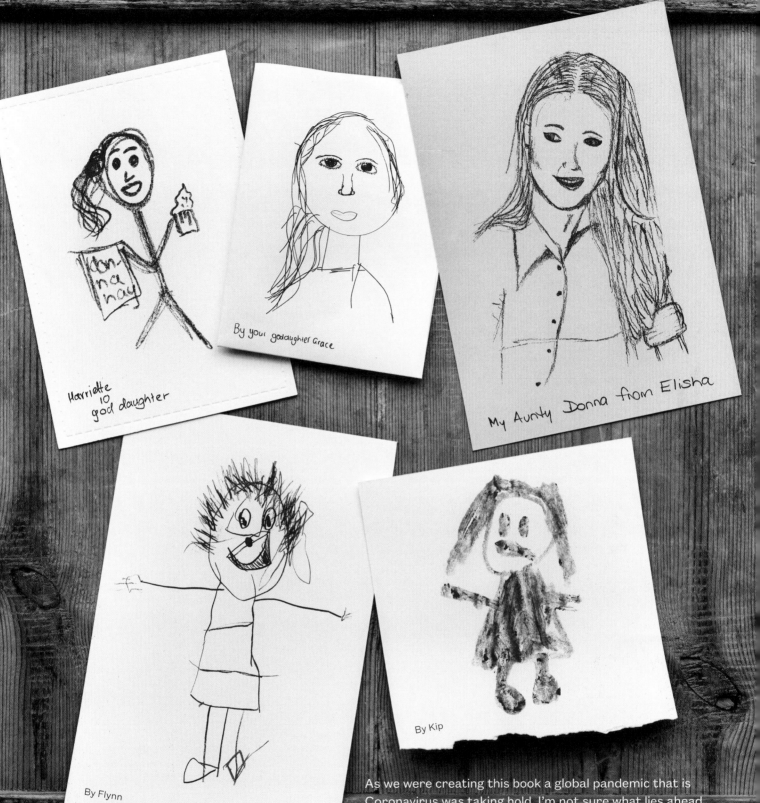

Harriette
10
god daughter

By your godaughter Grace

My Aunty Donna from Elisha

By Flynn

By Kip

As we were creating this book a global pandemic that is Coronavirus was taking hold. I'm not sure what lies ahead as businesses shut down and we work remotely to finish the book. All I know is that it's never been more important to look after and nourish our bodies, be kind to each other and to our world. I always leave my portrait to the end – this time it was too late! So I asked some special little friends who were staying safe at home to draw a portrait of me instead. I think these say it all and more! Dx

About
DONNA

As Australia's *leading food editor and bestselling cookbook author*, Donna Hay has made her way into hearts (and nearly every home) across the country.

An international publishing phenomenon, Donna's name is synonymous with accessible yet INSPIRATIONAL RECIPES and stunning images. Her acclaimed magazine notched up an incredible 100 issues and her bestselling cookbooks have sold more than *seven million copies worldwide*.

The donna hay brand goes beyond the printed page, featuring an *impressive digital presence*; a number of television series; branded merchandise; and a baking mix range in Australian supermarkets.

Donna is the very proud mum of two teenage boys, adores living near the ocean and still loves cooking every single day.